GLUCOSE HOMEOSTASIS

Edited by **Leszek Szablewski**

Glucose Homeostasis
http://dx.doi.org/10.5772/57190
Edited by Leszek Szablewski

Contributors

Robert Augustin, Aleksandra Zebrowska, Andrea M. P. Romani, Chesinta Voma, Ruben Marin-Juez, Francisco Carvalho-Simoes, Encarnación Capilla, Marta Camps, Josep V. Planas, Dayea Kim, Jong Hyuk Yoon, Jaeyoon Kim, Sung Ho Ryu, Menizibeya Welcome O., Lu Guang Luo, John YZ Luo, Souriya Vang, Ivor Jackson, Ting Zhao

Published by InTech

Janeza Trdine 9, 51000 Rijeka, Croatia

Publishing Process Manager Iva Lipovic

Technical Editor InTech DTP team

Cover InTech Design team

First published June, 2014

Printed in Croatia

Additional hard copies can be obtained from orders@intechopen.com

Glucose Homeostasis, Edited by Leszek Szablewski

p. cm.

ISBN 978-953-51-1618-9

For EU product safety concerns:
IN TECH d.o.o., Prolaz Marije Krucifikse Kozulić 3, 51000 Rijeka, Croatia,
info@intechopen.com or visit our website at intechopen.com.

Meet the editor

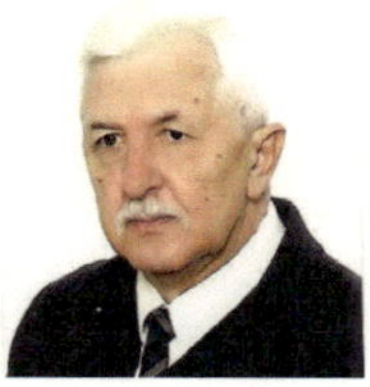

Dr. Leszek Szablewski graduated from University of Warsaw, Poland. He received his M.S. degree in Faculty of Biology from the same University. He obtained his Ph. D. from Institute of Experimental Biology Polish Academy of Sciences and habilitated in Medical University of Warsaw. Dr. Szablewski has experience in cell physiology, genetics and pathophysiology. He works on damages of glucose uptake and expression of glucose transporters in peripheral blood cells due to diabetes mellitus (in dependence on mode of therapy), surgical procedures and selected tumor cells. He previously worked with Tetrahymena pyriformis and T. rostrata (Ciliata) as a model of animal cell.

Contents

Preface

At least one in ten people today are destined, on current trends, to develop diabetes at some point during their lifetime. The total number of individuals with diabetes worldwide is scheduled to double in a generation. WHO has defined type 2 diabetes mellitus, a progressive worldwide epidemic. The statistics are alarming: 30 million people were diagnosed with diabetes worldwide in 1985. By 1995, the number had risen to 135 million. It has been estimated that by 2010, 220 million people worldwide will be affected by the disease, and there will be some 300 million by the year 2015 as predicted by WHO. According to another statistics, the prevalence of all forms of diabetes is estimated to be 2–3% of the world's population, with the number of diabetic patients increasing by 4–5% per annum. Moreover, many people with diabetes remain undiagnosed.

Type 1 diabetes is observed in approximately 5–10% of patients with diabetes mellitus. The incidence of type 1 diabetes is projected to increase 40% between 1997 and 2010. The studies suggest an annual global increase of 3–4% with the highest increase expected in the 0–4 year age group.

The progress in molecular biology, genetics, epidemiology and in clinical applications notwithstanding, much more needs to be done. It will be of great importance to identify the molecular mechanisms of diabetes and insulin resistance.

Most tissues and organs, such as the brain, need glucose constantly, as an important source of energy. The low blood concentrations of glucose can cause seizures, loss of consciousness, and death. On the other hand, long lasting elevation of blood glucose concentrations can result in blindness, renal failure, cardiac and peripheral vascular disease, and neuropathy. Therefore, blood glucose concentrations need to be maintained within narrow limits. The process of maintaining blood glucose at a steady-state level is called glucose homeostasis. This is accomplished by the finely hormone regulation of peripheral glucose uptake (glucose utilization), hepatic glucose production and glucose uptake during carbohydrates ingestion.

Glucose is obtained directly from the diet and by the synthesis from other substances in organs such as liver. Glucose derived from the diet is transferred from the lumen of small intestine, and both dietary glucose and glucose synthesized within the body have to be transported from the circulation into target cell. Glucose cannot penetrate the lipid bilayer, and specific carrier proteins are required to its diffusion. These transporters comprise two structurally and functionally distinct groups, whose members have been identified over the past decades, namely: the Na^+-dependent co-transporter (SGLT) and the facilitative, Na^+-independent sugar transporters (GLUT). These various transporters exhibit different substrate specificities, kinetic properties and tissue expression profiles.

The book entitled "Glucose Homeostasis" edited by Dr. Leszek Szablewski provides a broad overview of the molecular, biochemical, and clinical aspects of glucose metabolism, insulin resistance and diabetes mellitus. The chapters will make the reader acquainted with a variety of topics ranging from glucose transporters, glucose homeostasis and influence of adipokines and TRH on cells. This book is written by authors from different laboratories, yet, the editor has tried to arrange the book chapters in a single volume to make it easier for the readers to find what they need.

Section 1, which includes chapters 1-2, mainly describes the Na^+-dependent co-transporter (SGLT) and facilitative, Na^+-independent glucose transporters (GLUT) and the important role of GLUT 4 in glucose homeostasis.

Section 2, which includes chapters 3-5, describes the mechanisms of glucose homeostasis.

Section 3, which includes chapters 6-7, describes the influence of adipokines and TRH on cells.

This book will be of help to scientists, doctors, pharmacists, and other experts in various disciplines.

Dr. Leszek Szablewski
Chair of General Biology & Parasitology
Center of Biostructure Research
Medical University of Warsaw
Poland

Section 1

Glucose Transporters

Chapter 1

Mammalian Sugar Transporters

Robert Augustin and Eric Mayoux

Additional information is available at the end of the chapter

http://dx.doi.org/10.5772/58325

1. Introduction

Glucose represents the major energy source of mammalian cells. Due to its hydrophilic nature, glucose requires specific transporters in order to cross cellular membranes. Such transport is, in the case of glucose and also other monosaccharides, mediated by energy-coupled as well as facilitative mechanisms represented by protein families of sodium-driven sugar cotransporters (SGLTs) and glucose transporters (GLUTs), respectively.

SGLT cotransporter family present highly diverse functions. They cotransport Na+ with glucose (SGLT1, SGLT2, SGLT4, SGLT5), or galactose (SGLT1, SGLT5) or mannose (SGLT5) or fructose (SGLT5) but also with myoinositol (SGLT6, SMIT), with iodine (NIS) or with choline (CHT). One family member is not a transporter but a glucose sensor (SGLT3). Na+ gradient for this cotransporter family is maintained by Na+/K(+)-ATPase [1].

The various members of the GLUT protein family is comprised of 14 isoforms [2]

The GLUT protein family consists of three different families that can be distinguished based on their protein sequence homologies: Class I comprises the classical transporters GLUT1-4 as well as the gene duplication of GLUT3 which is GLUT14, Class II contains the isoforms GLUT5, 7, 9, and 11, while GLUT6, 8, 10, 12 and the proton-driven myo-inositol transporter HMIT (GLUT13) belong to the Class III [3].

Current understanding of whole body glucose homeostasis under normal-and, more importantly, under disease conditions-is directly linked to the understanding of SGLT and GLUT physiology (Figure 1). The active mechanism of glucose (as well as galactose) absorption in the intestine is primarily catalysed by SGLT1 (Figure 3B), while SGLT2 represents the predominant mechanism for glucose reuptake by the kidney (Figure 3A).

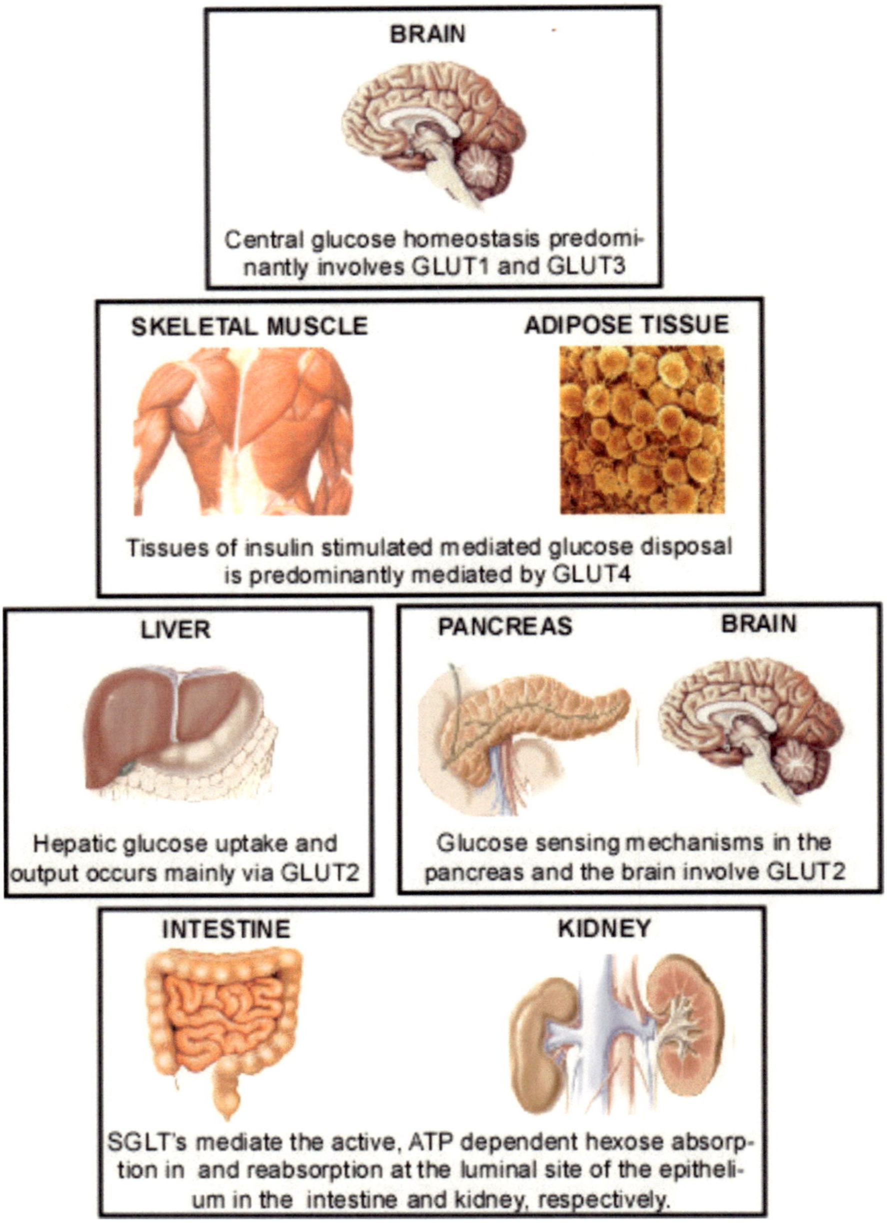

Figure 1. Overview on the principle physiological role for specific glucose transporters and their involvement in regulating glucose homeostasis in specific tissues.

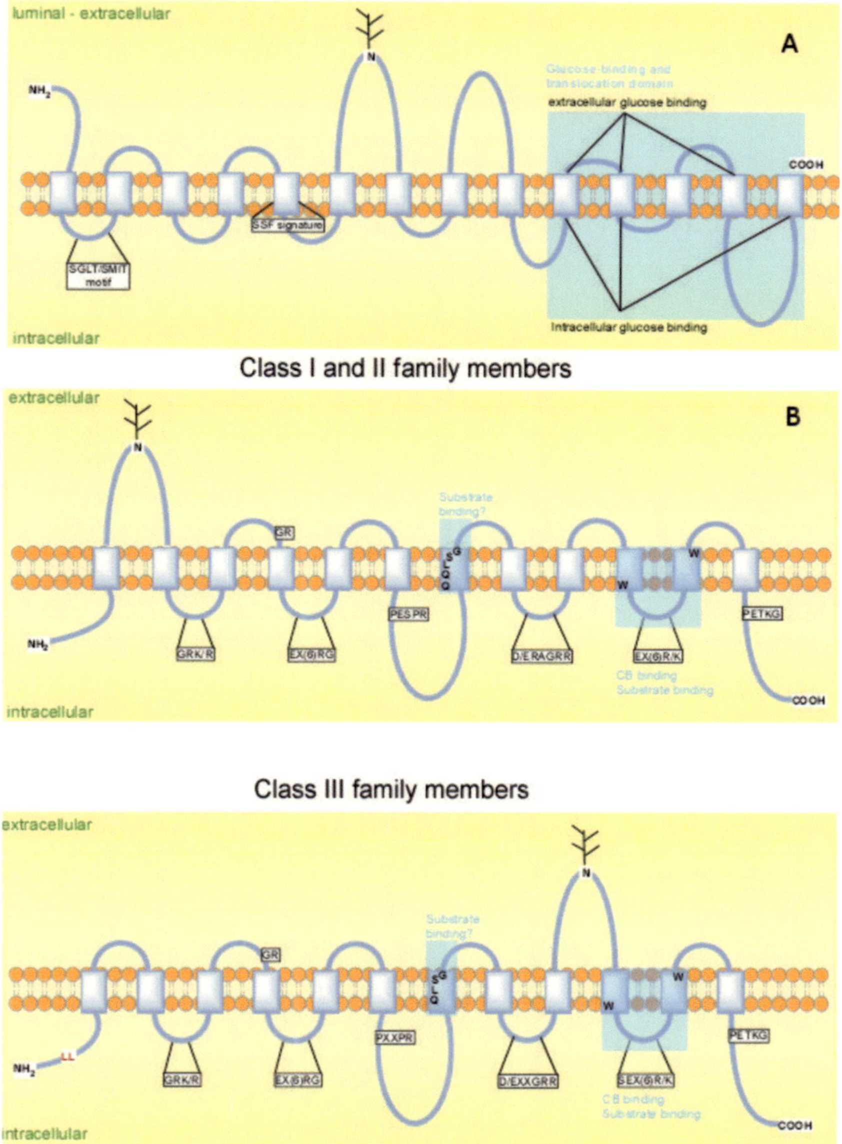

Figure 2. Putative secondary structural models for GLUT and SGLT proteins. **A-**SGLT family members contain 14 transmembrane domains [21]. Highlighted is the presence of the SSF motif present in all members of the solute symporter family (SSF) gene family. The motif that is shared between the SGLTs and sodium-myoinositol cotransporters (SMITs) is also indicated. The glucose-binding and-translocation domain is located at the COOH-terminus of the protein. The residues that are proposed to be involved in glucose binding at the extra-and intracellular sides of the membrane are highlighted. **B-**GLUT proteins contain 12 transmembrane regions. Specific structural features for class I and II (upper panel) and class III (lower panel) family members are indicated such as the proposed substrate binding site, the N-linked glycosylation sites, conserved signature sequences. The tryptophan residues implicated in cyto-chalasin B (CB) binding (positions 338 and 412 in GLUT1) and the N-terminal dileucine signal present in class III members (except for GLUT10) are also shown.

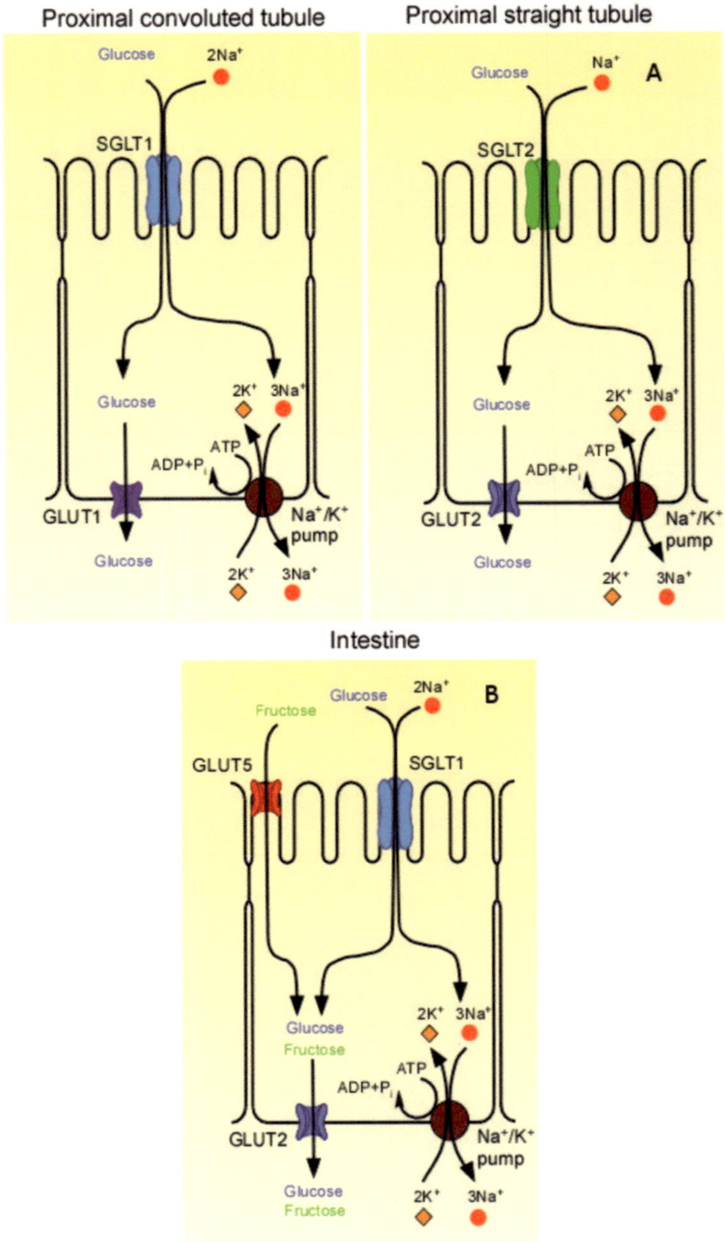

Figure 3. SGLT and GLUT family members regulate intestinal absorption and renal reabsorption of hexoses.A-Renal glucose reabsorption. In the kidney, proximal tubule transepithelial reabsorption of glucose occurs at the apical membrane by SGLT2 and GLUT2 at the basolateral membrane. In the proximal straight tubule, the remaining glucose is reabsorbed by SGLT1 at the apical site of the epithelium and GLUT1 at the basolateral membrane. **B-Intestinal glucose absorption.** In the intestine, transepithelial glucose uptake at the apical site is mediated by the Na^+-dependent glucose transporter SGLT1, while fructose is absorbed by facilitated diffusion via GLUT5. These hexoses can all exit the basolateral membrane through GLUT2.

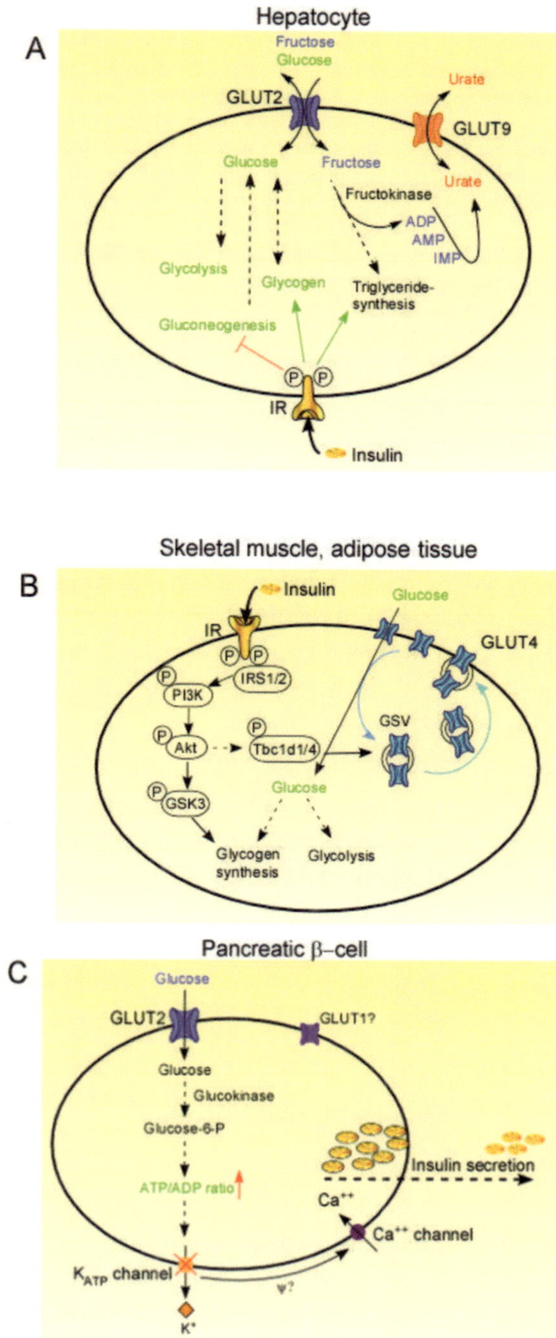

Figure 4. GLUT family members facilitate glucose transport into tissues that control glucose homeostasis such as hepatocytes, skeletal muscle, adipose tissue, and the pancreatic β-cells of the islets of Langerhans. A-Hexose transport in hepatocytes. GLUT2 mediates glucose uptake under feeding conditions into hepatocytes where glucose is metabolized by glycolysis or incorporated into glycogen. In patients with FBS fructose handling is normal, therefore

GLUT2 might not be exclusively involved in uptake of this ketohexose by the hepatocyte [38]. GLUT9 is highly expressed in liver and due to its capability to transport uric acid its proposed function in humans might be the release of uric acid from the liver. In mice GLUT9 is required for uric acid uptake into liver for further breakdown by uricase to allantoin [39]. Whether GLUT9 also contributes to hexose transport, namely fructose, in hepatocytes is currently unknown. Fructose that is taken up by the liver mainly feeds into triglyceride synthesis, and via ATP depletion stimulates AMP-deaminase and thereby purine degradation leading to an increased generation of uric acid. **B-Insulin stimulated glucose uptake into skeletal muscle and adipose tissue**. In muscle and fat, glucose uptake is stimulated by insulin. After insulin binds to its receptor, auto-phosphorylation of the receptor occurs that triggers a signalling cascade that finally leads to a translocation of GLUT4 vesicles from an intracellular pool to the plasma membrane. The acute increase of GLUT4 molecules at the cell surface leads to an increase in glucose uptake and represents the rate-limiting step in insulin-stimulated glucose uptake in adipose and muscle tissues. **C-Pancreatic β-cells secrete insulin in response to elevations in blood glucose**. GLUT2 mediates glucose uptake into β-cells. Phosphorylation of glucose by glucokinase is the rate limiting step of glycolysis which increases the ATP to ADP ratio of the cell leading to closure of the K_{ATP} channel and subsequent opening of the of Ca^{++}channels caused presumably by changes of the plasma membrane polarization. The opening of Ca^{++}channels raises intracellular Ca^{++}concentrations and induces exocytosis of the insulin granules.

As the brain's main energy source glucose needs to be transported across the blood-brain barrier. This process is facilitated by GLUT1 (Figure 1). Insulin-stimulated clearance of blood glucose through uptake into skeletal muscle, the heart and adipose tissue, the rate-limiting step is defined by translocation of GLUT4 from an intracellular compartment to the plasma membrane; and it's this signalling cascade that represents insulin sensitivity (Figure 4B). The secretion of insulin by the pancreatic β-cells of the islets of Langerhans is dependent on GLUT2 which functions as a β-cell glucose sensor (Figure 4C). However, the involvement of sugar transporters in the regulation of processes such as brain glucose sensing or glucose transport in the mammary gland are not yet well understood.

This chapter summarizes the principal characteristics of SGLT [1] and GLUT-[4] mediated sugar transport, primarily focusing on the human transporters, with emphasis on the current understanding of their physiology, based on inherited disorders and syndromes in humans and phenotypes of genetically modified mice.

2. The SGLT family

2.1. Synonyms

SGLT1-6, Gene Symbols: *SLC5*, sodium-glucose symporters

2.2. Summary

The model of active, ATP-dependent glucose transport against a concentration gradient was proposed in 1960 by Bob Crane [5]. Intestinal reabsorption of glucose by the intestinal epithelium through transporters requires sodium symport which is ATP dependent via coupling to the sodium/potassium (Na^+/K^+) pump. Mechanistically, the inward sodium gradient at the apical site of epithelial cells is maintained by the ATP-driven, active extrusion of sodium at the basolateral membrane (Figure 3, Figure 5B). The sodium dependent glucose transporters (SGLTs) are members of a larger gene family (>200 genes) of sodium:solute symporters (SSF) that contain a common SSF motif in the fifth transmembrane region [1]. The

http://dx.doi.org/10.5772/58325

human SGLT protein family (SLC5A) comprises 11 isoforms that structurally are characterized by 14 transmembrane domains, where the N-and C-termini face the extracellular (luminal) side of the cell. The 11 family members share an amino acid identity of 21-70%. A broad range of substrates are transported by proteins encoded by the *SLC5* genes.

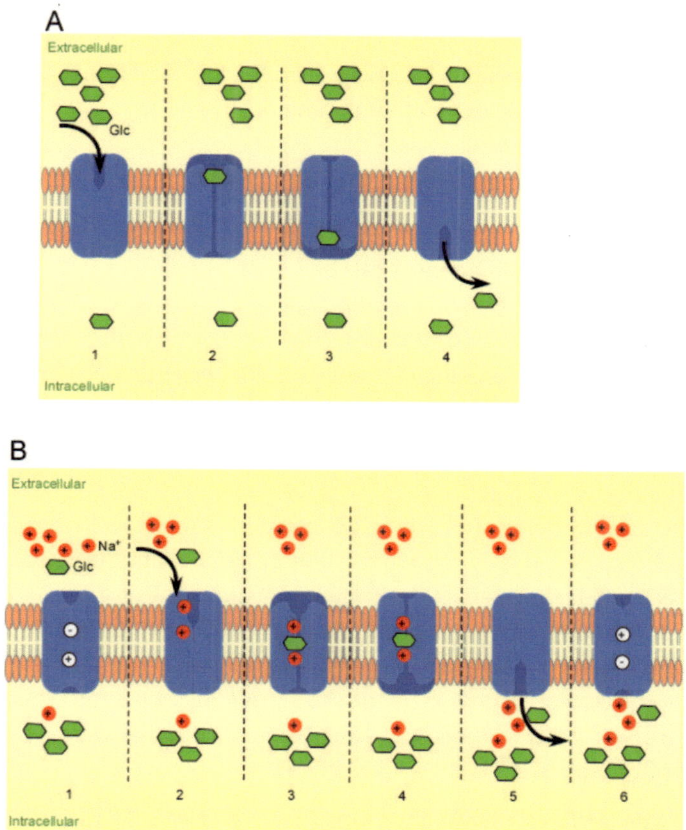

Figure 5. Proposed models for the mechanism of facilitative and active glucose transport across cellular membranes.A-A 6-state model is proposed for SGLT mediated glucose transport. The empty transporter is assumed to have a valence of-2 (1). Sugar transport is initiated upon binding of two sodium ions to the open form of the outside gate (2). In the next step, glucose binds to the transporter, which induces a conformational change from an outward to an inward occluded state (3, 4). Upon open of the inward gate, the glucose is released into the cytoplasm before the sodium (5). The transport cycle is completed by a conformational change to return the ligand-free inward facing (6) structure to the ligand-free outward-facing structure (1). **B-Model of GLUT mediated glucose transport.** Glucose binds to an outward-facing site of the transporter (1) which induces a conformational changes that allows movement of the hexose through the protein (2-3). After the release of the hexose from its inward-facing binding site into the cytosol the transporter undergoes a reverse conformational change (4-1).

The focus of the current chapter is on the sodium-dependent glucose transporters within the *SLC5* gene family, namely SGLT1-5, and the closely related, based on sequence homology and substrate specificity, sodium driven myoinositol transporter SMIT1 (SLC5A3) and SMIT2 (SGLT6/SLC5A11).

More distant relatives of the *SLC5A* gene family are the iodide transporters NIS (sodium-iodide symporter [SLC5A5]) and AIT (apical iodide transporter [SLC5A11]), the Na+/Cl-/choline transporter (CHT, [SLC5A7]) and the sodium-dependent multivitamin transporter (SMVT, [SLC5A6]). NIS and AIT are expressed in the thyroid gland. While NIS is responsible for iodide uptake which is required for production of T3 and T4, AIT is thought to catalyse the movement of iodide from the thyrocyte cytoplasm to the lumen of the gland. SMVT is widely expressed, while

CHT is mainly found in the central nervous system. Biochemically, the CHT mediates Na+/ choline co-transport in a chloride dependent manner.

2.3. Structural features & substrate specificities

SGLT family members 1-6 contain between 596-681 amino acids with a 50-70% identity (67-84% similarity) where divergence in sequences can be mainly attributed to the N-and C-terminal domains of the proteins. Alternative splicing has been described for SGLT4-6, however, whether respective functional proteins with varying amino acid composition are encoded has yet to be shown. A common structural component among the large gene family of sodium:solute symporters (SSF) is the presence of a consensus pattern (Figure 2A). The consensus sequence for the six SGLTs and for SMIT1 is located near the N-terminal domain of the proteins (Figure 2A).

A secondary structural model for human SGLT1 predicts the presence of 14 transmembrane helices. The model is based on N-glycosylation and cysteine scanning mutagenesis, antibody tagging, mass spectrometry as well as computer algorithms predicting membrane-spanning regions (Figure 2A). Freeze-fracture electron microscopy provided direct evidence that both SGLT1 and vSGLT (from *Vibrio parahaemolyticus*) function as 14 transmembrane helical monomers. he recent crystal structure for the sodium/galactose symporter vSGLT demonstrated the presence of 14 transmembrane helices providing evidence for the secondary structural model of human SGLT1.

SGLT are highly glycosylated membrane proteins for example SGLT1 contains a N-linked glycosylation site at position N248. However, for SGLT1, glycosylation appears not to be required for functional expression, indicating proper folding and membrane targeting in its absence.

The transport kinetics and substrate specificities have been intensively studied for SGLT1, 2, 3, and more recently 4, mainly based on electrophysiological and biochemical studies upon heterologous expression of the transporters in *Xenopus laevis* oocytes. SGLT1-4 and SMIT1 and 2 all transport (or bind in the case of human SGLT3) D-glucose and the non-metabolizable alpha-methyl-d-glucopyranoside (α-DMG). Transport of those substrates is inhibited by the glycoside phlorizin [6].

SGLT are only able to transport sugars with a pyranose ring, cyclic polyhydroxy alcohols are not transported. The importance of the single hydroxyl groups for substrate recognition has been well characterized. The oxygen is essential for transport by human SGLT1-while sulfur substitution lowers affinity, nitrogen is not tolerated. This particular feature does not apply to

SGLT3 for which imino sugars-containing an amine group in place of a hydroxyl group-are ligands. Based on mutational analysis of SGLTs and the crystal structure of vSGLT, which is 32% identical to human SGLT1, residues that coordinate substrate recognition have been shown to be relatively conserved. An exception to that is the human SGLT3, a glucose sensor, which can be converted to a functional transporter based on a single amino acid exchange.

In addition to glucose and other monosaccharides, SGLTs also transport glycosides. Those can be either substrates such as indican and arbutin, or actual inhibitors such as the highly potent, classic competitive SGLT inhibitor phlorizin, a naturally occurring β-glucoside (see below).

The ability to recognize galactose as substrate by SLC5 family members has been attributed to the presence of a threonine corresponding to amino acid 460 in human SGLT1.

Ion selectivity and stoichiometry has been well characterized for SGLTs. The transporters are selective for the cotransport cation Na^+(K_m=4mM). While Li^+(K_m=9mM) and H^+(K_m=7μM) can replace Na^+, no other monovalent cation is accepted. The Na^+ to glucose transport stoichiometry is established for SGLT1-3, where two Na^+ ions bind to SGLT1 and 3, and only one Na^+ is required to drive SGLT2 activity. Despite crystallographic information for vSGLT, the electron density is not sufficient to assign binding sites for small single ions such as sodium. However, using mutational analysis and superimposition of structural models from the solute symporters vSGLT, LeuT, and Mhp1, a sodium binding site for vSGLT is suggested to be close to the sugar binding residues in transmembrane domains 1 and 8. The predicted cation binding site in vSGLT appears to allow accessibility to the cytoplasmic aqueous phase.

The mechanism of sodium-driven glucose transport has been intensively investigated for SGLT1, applying various methodologies that allow the kinetics of transport to be determined using heterologous expression of the transporter in *Xenopus laevis* oocytes. From the kinetic measurements a 6-state equilibrium model is proposed, where conformational changes dependent on cation and sugar binding, transport and cytoplasmic release are integrated. The six kinetic states describe the "empty" transporter, the sodium bound form, and the sodium and glucose bound transporter at the external and internal plasma membrane surfaces (Figure 5A).

SGLT1 mediated glucose transport has been characterized regarding its kinetics, conformational changes and the significance of residues for substrate/inhibitor binding. However, many questions remain unanswered such as the precise identity of the second-sodium binding site for SGLT1, and the location of the phlorizin binding site in SGLT1 and SGLT2, which may be of relevance for SGLT2 selective inhibitors that, recently approved, represent a new treatment option for Type 2 diabetes mellitus (T2DM) (see below).

2.4. SGLT1 (*SLC5A1*)

In 1987, the laboratory of Ernest Wright cloned the first sodium-dependent glucose transporter from rabbit intestinal mRNA by an expressing cloning strategy using *Xenopus laevis* oocytes [1]. SGLT1 is primarily expressed in the brush border membrane of mature enterocytes in the small intestine and catalyses the absorption of the dietary sugars glucose and galactose from the gut lumen. SGLT1 is also expressed in the kidney on the luminal surface of cells within the S3 segment of the proximal tubule, where it contributes to renal glucose reabsorption (Figure 3A).

SGLT1 is a high-affinity, low-capacity transporter with a K_m of 0.5 mM for the substrate αMDG in *Xenopus laevis* oocytes. Substrate transport of glucose is coupled to symport of two sodium ions. The protein is highly glycosylated which leads to an apparent molecular weight of 75 kDa.

2.4.1. SGLT1 physiology

Humans with deficiency for SGLT1 display glucose and galactose malabsorption

Mutations in the SGLT1 gene cause glucose-galactose malabsorption (GGM). GGM was first described in 1962 [7] as a severe life-threatening diarrhea in new-born children, that is fatal within weeks unless lactose, glucose, and galactose are removed from the diet. The diarrhea returns immediately upon reintroduction of the respective sugars into the diet. GGM was predicted to be caused by defective intestinal sodium-coupled glucose transport, a hypothesis that was confirmed following the cloning of human SGLT1 and the identification of homozygous carriers for the D28N mutation encoding a non-functional protein [8].

GGM is a rare autosomal recessive disease caused by missense, nonsense, frame-shift, and splice-site mutations within the SGLT1 gene. Missense mutations-even single amino acid changes-have been demonstrated to cause missorting of the protein in cells, suggesting that slight conformational changes in the protein can interfere with proper folding and/or delivery and integration of SGLT1 into the plasma membrane and thereby affecting its function. More than 80 patients with GGM have been screened for mutations in the SGLT1 gene [1].

2.5. SGLT2 (*SLC5A2)*

SGLT2 was cloned from human kidney cDNA in 1992 and was found to encode for a 672 amino acid protein with 59% similarity to SGLT1. SGLT2 is almost exclusively expressed in the kidney and localizes to the apical domain of epithelial cells that line the S1/S2 segments of the proximal convoluted renal tubule. It has been characterized as a kidney-specific transporter controlling the initial step of renal glucose reabsorption, working in concert with SGLT1, which appears responsible for clearance of residual glucose in the more distal S3 segment of the proximal tubular system (Figure 3A). In contrast to SGLT1, which transports glucose and galactose, SGLT2 represents a low-affinity, high-capacity sodium-glucose symporter with a K_m for glucose of 6 mM and a sodium-to-glucose coupling ratio of 1:1 while having no affinity for galactose.

2.5.1. SGLT2 physiology

Human Physiology-Familial Renal Glucosuria (FRG) is caused by non-functional SGLT2

Glucosuria in the absence of both generalized proximal tubular dysfunction and hyperglycemia is known as De-Toni-Debré-Fanconi syndrome. This is recognized as an inherited disorder and designated as familial renal glucosuria (FRG).

FRG is an autosomal recessive disorder and is diagnosed by persistent isolated glucosuria (urine excretion >1 g/day) with normal fasting plasma glucose levels and oral glucose tolerance.

Since the first SLC5A2 mutation in FRG was presented in 2002 [9], forty-four mutations have been identified including premature stops, frame shifts, and missense mutations. Although the pattern of inheritance for FRG is of co-dominance, a clear definition of genotype-phenotype correlation has not been established. Individuals with similar or even identical mutations display a broad range of severity in glucosuria, indicating that environmental, as well as genetic, factors affect urinary glucose reabsorption. Since, thus far, none of the FRG mutations has been tested for functional SGLT2 effects it is unknown how the various mutations relate to the severity of glucosuria.

FRG established the fundamental role of SGLT2 in renal glucose reabsorption. Since patients with FRG are not affected by severe clinical consequences, it is considered a benign condition, more a phenotype than a disease.

Mouse models of SGLT2 deficiency

The metabolic consequences of SGLT2 deficiency in mice have been investigated in a model of diet-induced obesity and associated insulin resistance and a genetic model of T2DM, the db/db mouse strain [10]. Deletion of SGLT2 leads to increased urine output and a tremendous increase in glucosuria that is associated with compensatory increases in feeding, drinking, and activity. SGLT2 knockout mice are protected from diet-induced hyperglycemia and glucose intolerance and have reduced plasma insulin concentrations. In the diabetic db/db mouse, deficiency of SGLT2 prevents fasting hyperglycemia and is associated with normalized plasma insulin levels and preserved pancreatic β-cell function. These data confirm the concept of glucotoxicity which was established by studying the anti-diabetic effects of blocking renal glucose reabsorption in diabetic rats by pharmacological means of SGLT inhibition using phlorizin [11].

2.5.2. SGLT2 inhibitors – A new concept for the treatment of Type 2 diabetes

T2DM is characterized by hyperglycemia that results both from peripheral resistance to the action of insulin and from progressive failure of the pancreatic β-cell to compensate for the increasing demand for insulin. Chronic hyperglycemia triggers glucotoxicity, a term summarizing the vicious cycle between hyperglycemia inducing β-cell dysfunction and insulin resistance that aggravates disease progression leading to micro-and macrovascular complications.

Current treatments for T2DM come with significant limitations regarding their potential to induce adverse effects. Metformin can cause gastrointestinal effects such as diarrhea and nausea, while sulfonylureas and insulin can induce hypoglycemia and are associated with weight gain. Thiazolidinediones that act as insulin sensitizers can induce weight gain, and are associated with edema and are potentially associated with an increased cardiovascular risk. GLP-1 analogues which are incretin mimicking agents can cause nausea and diarrhea. New therapeutic strategies are needed that are not only effective in terms of glucose control, but provide excellent safety and potential add-on effects such as weight loss, lipid lowering or reductions in blood pressure.

The kidney has an important role in controlling blood glucose levels by mediating glucose reabsorption into the bloodstream. In patients with T2DM increased renal absorptive capacity has been observed, indicating that blocking the process of glucose reuptake by the kidney might be an attractive new strategy for treatment of T2DM. However, glucosuria has historically been perceived as a manifestation of the disease, which appears to make this therapeutic concept seem rather counter-intuitive.

The phenotype of subjects identified with FRG, as well as studies performed with phlorizin, indicated that correcting hyperglycemia via specific inhibition of SGLT2 might provide a new option for a safe and effective treatment of T2DM.

Phlorizin, a potent SGLT inhibitor, proved to be an important tool for investigating the mechanism and consequences of blocking renal sugar reabsorption. Its use established the concept of glucotoxicity: blocking of renal glucose reabsorption with phlorizin in diabetic rats normalized insulin levels and restored insulin sensitivity [11].

Disadvantages of phlorizin include the non-selective inhibition of SGLT2, poor bioavailability, short half-life and potential for side effects caused e.g by blocking GLUT via its major metabolite phloretin. These disadvantages that are inherited to the molecular phlorizin led into research for new compounds in order to achieve proof of concept for selective SGLT2 inhibition for the treatment of T2DM.

Although non-selective for SGLT2, T-1095 was the first orally available phlorizin derivative that was metabolically stable. When administered to diabetic animals, T-1095 corrected hyperglycemia and reduced hyperinsulinemia, and hypertriglyceridemia [12]. These findings indicated that SGLT2 inhibition might be a viable approach to treatment of T2DM.

In the following years, the selective SGLT2 inhibitors sergliflozin and remogliflozin progressed to clinical trials. While many selective SGLT2 inhibitors went into clinical testing, development of O-glycosidic SGLT2 inhibitors was halted, presumably due to their unfavorable pharmakokinetic profile. In contrast, a number of C-glycosidic compounds which differ from O-glycosides in structure and stability are in clinical development [12] or have achieved approval and represent an innovative insulin-independent treatment option for controlling blood glucose in Type 2 diabetic patients [13].

2.6. SGLT3 (*SLC5A4*)

The human SGLT3 cDNA was cloned from colon carcinoma and was found to encode a 659 amino acid protein with 70% identity to human SGLT1. SGLT3 mRNA is detected in the intestine, testes, uterus, lung, brain and thyroid, while the protein is predominantly found in intestine and skeletal muscle. Immunohistochemical analysis of the intestine identified cholinergic neurons in submucosal and myenteric plexuses as the site of SGLT3 expression. In skeletal muscle, SGLT3 co-localized with the nicotinic acetylcholine receptor indicating expression at the neuromuscular junction.

Functional characterization of human SGLT3 demonstrated a lack of sugar transport activity. Instead, human SGLT3 was found to be a glucose-sensitive ion channel where sugar binding induces plasma membrane depolarization in a saturable, sodium-dependent and phlorizin-sensitive manner [14]. Interestingly, this is in sharp contrast to pig and mouse SGLT3 which are able to transport glucose. The sodium-to-substrate stoichiometry is 2:1, which is similar to SGLT1, while substrate specificity appears closer to SGLT2 with no acceptance of galactose as a substrate. More in depth characterization of SGLT3 substrate specifities found that human SGLT3, similarly to SGLT1, interacts with various glucosides, while pig SGLT3 was found to transport imino sugars with high affinity.

The lack of transport activity by human SGLT3 has been shown to involve a specific amino acid: residue 457. This residue has been shown to be important for the function of human SGLT1, since mutations of that particular amino acid cause GGM. Structural information from vSGLT [15] revealed that the corresponding residue mediates direct interaction with the sugar. Accordingly, mutation of glutamate 457 in human SGLT3 to glutamine conferred transport activity on the transporter displaying SGLT1-like transport characteristics with respect to substrate-to-sodium stoichiometry, sugar specificities as well as affinities [15].

Physiologically, SGLT3 is hypothesized to act as a glucose sensor which, at the site of its expression in cholinergic neurons and the neuromuscular junction, might modulate action potentials of neurons/skeletal muscle cells glucose dependently. This hypothesis is supported by the observation that upon expression of human SGLT3 in sensory neurons of *C. elegans* glucose sensing *in vivo* can be monitored [16]. More recent observations indicated that SGLT3 is expressed in the proximal tubule of the human kidney and might be responsible for sodium reabsorption based on uptake studies in SGLT3 overexpressing kidney cell lines which demonstrated sodium transport that was blocked by the classical inhibitor phlorizin [17].

2.7. SGLT4 (*SLC5A9*)

SGLT4 was cloned from human small intestinal cDNA libraries. The mRNA encoding SGLT4 is almost exclusively found in the small intestine and kidney. SGLT4 exhibits Na+-dependent AMG transport with a K_m of 2.6 mM. Inhibition studies of AMG mediated transport indicated that SGLT4 appears to transport naturally occurring sugars with a rank order of mannose, glucose, fructose, and galactose. Transport studies using radiolabeled mannose indicated that SGLT4 might be physiologically relevant for intestinal absorption as well as renal reabsorption of mannose [18].

2.8. SGLT5 (*SLC5A10*)

SGLT5 was recently cloned from human kidney cDNA and characterized as a kidney specific sodium-dependent mannose transporter which is also able to transport glucose and fructose [19]. While specifically expressed in human kidney its precise localization and physiological role remains unknown. Based on amino acid sequence homology SGLT5 represents the closest homologue to SGLT4. In a manner reminiscent of the relationship between SGLT1 and SGLT2, it can be speculated that SGLT4 and SGLT5 may act as complementary mannose transporters that regulate intestinal absorption and renal reabsorption of mannose, respectively.

Mouse models of SGLT5 deficiency

Mice deficient for SGLT5 [20] were shown not to display any renal sodium-dependent fructose uptake but increased urinary fructose indicating that SGLT5 is the major transporter responsible for fructose reabsorption in the kidney. Fructose consumption especially by corn syrup containing beverages has been epidemiologically linked to dyslipidemia, obesity, and diabetes. Despite its role in renal fructose reuptake, knockout of SGLT5 in mice paradoxically exacerbated fructose-induced hepatic steatosis.

The massive urinary fructose excretion was accompanied by reduced levels of plasma triglycerides and epididymal fat but fasting hyperinsulinemia. No difference in food consumption, water intake, or plasma fructose was described for SGLT5 deficient mice. The phenotype of SGLT5 knockout mice indicated an apparent link between renal fructose reabsorption and hepatic lipid metabolism.

2.9. SMIT1 (*SLC5A3*)

A Na(+)/myoinositol cotransporter cDNA (SLC5A3) was cloned from canine renal cells and sequenced in 1992 followed by the human SLC5A3 in 1995. The human transporter is mainly expressed in kidney, brain, placenta, pancreas, heart, skeletal muscle, and the lung.

2.9.1. SMIT1 physiology

Phenotype of mice deficient for SMIT1

Myoinositol is a precursor of the main inositol-containing phospholipids phosphatidylinositol and phosphatidylinositol-4,5-bisphosphate, a key molecule in cellular signal transduction. In addition, myoinositol has an important role in osmoregulation. The highest myoinositol levels are found in certain regions of the brain with cerebrospinal fluid levels ranging from 2-25 mM, which are higher than levels in the blood.

One hypothesis as to why lithium is effective in the treatment of bipolar disorders is based on its effect on reducing cellular concentrations of myoinositol (the inositol depletion model). Ablation of the murine *SLC5A3* gene demonstrated the significant role of this transporter in maintaining central myoinositol concentrations. SMIT1 knockout mice have significantly reduced central inositol levels with no changes in phosphatidylinositol concentrations. Besides the severe myoinositol deficiency in the brain, those animals display congenital central apnea due to abnormal respiratory rhythmogenesis leading to death shortly after birth. The neonatal lethality of SMIT1 knockout animals appears to be caused by failures in development of peripheral nerves, specifically in nerves controlling breathing. The peripheral nerve abnormalities can be corrected by prenatal myoinositol supplementation suggesting that myoinositol is required for peripheral nerve development. Phenotypic analysis of homozygous SMIT1 knockout mice indicated, that a reduction of central inositol levels is associated with lithium-

http://dx.doi.org/10.5772/58325

like neurobehavioral effects. Potentially, the inositol depletion hypothesis as a mode of action for lithium might be supported by the phenotypic characteristics of SMIT1 knockout mice [21].

2.10. SGLT6 /SMIT2 (*SLC5A11*)

SMIT2 was initially cloned by PCR from rabbit kidney cDNA. Sequence analysis indicated 49% and 43% protein sequence identity to SGLT1 and SMIT1, respectively. SMIT2 mRNA is detected in brain, kidney, heart, skeletal muscle, spleen, liver, placenta, lung, leukocytes, and neurons. Three transcript variants named SMIT1a, SMIT1b, and SMIT1c have been identified for the *SLC5A2* gene. It wasn't until 2002, that the cloned product was functionally characterized and identified as a sodium-coupled myoinositol transporter with a K_m of 120 μM and 13 mM for myoinositol and sodium, respectively [22]. Transport mediated by SMIT2 is phlorizin sensitive (K_i of 76 μm). The substrate specificities of SMIT1 and SMIT2 are remarkably different: SMIT2 shows stereospecific transport of D-glucose and D-xylose without affinity for fucose, while SMIT1 transports L-fucose and L-xylose (but not their D-isomers) and does not distinguish between D-and L-glucose. In contrast to SMIT1, SMIT2 transports d-*chiro*-inositol.

SMIT2 mediated myo-inositol transport has been demonstrated to occur at apical membranes of the rat intestine [23] and at the luminal side of of proximal convoluted tubules in the kidney of rabbits [24], a tissue specificity and principle role that appears similar to the sodium-dependent uptake and reabsorption of glucose mediated by SGLT-1.

3. The family of glucose transport facilitators

3.1. Synonyms

GLUT1-14, Gene Symbols: *SLC2A1-14*, solute carrier family 2A1-14

3.2. Summary

Glucose transporters are uniporters that facilitate the diffusion of their respective substrates (e.g. glucose) across cellular membranes along a concentration gradient [2, 4]. The protein family comprises 14 isoforms that share common structural features such as 12 transmembrane domains, N-and C-termini facing the cytoplasm of the cell and an N-glycosylation site within either the first or fifth extracellular loop. Based on their sequence homology (14-63% identity) three classes can be distinguished: Class I includes the 'classic' glucose transporters GLUT1-4 and GLUT14, the Class II members are GLUT5, 7, 9, 11, and the Class III transporters comprise GLUT6, 8, 10, 12 and the proton driven myo-inositol transporter HMIT (or GLUT13). Despite their structural similarities, the different isoforms are characterized by tissue specific expression and distinct characteristics such as alternative splicing and (sub) cellular localization. With respect to their substrate specificities, the protein family includes transporters of glucose (GLUT1-4, 8, 14), fructose (GLUT5, 7, 11), polyol (GLUT12), myo-inositol (GLUT13), and urea (GLUT9) transporters.

More in-depth phylogenetic analysis of the GLUT sequences implied a different clustering of GLUT6 and 8, GLUT10 and GLUT12, and HMIT as more distant family members implying the existence of 5 subclasses based on sequence identities but in addition functional properties. Based on these analysis, the evolutionary more ancient forms HMIT, GLUT10, 12, 6, and 8 are postulated to mediate substrate transport which is linked to electrochemical gradients as it has been described for HMIT and GLUT12 [25].

3.3. Structural features & substrate specificity

The protein sequences of the 14 isoforms protein sequences are between 14-63% identical and 30-79% conserved. Common to all isoforms of the GLUT protein family are the predicted 12 transmembrane helices that are based on the initial hydropathy plot for GLUT1 (Figure 2B). The 12-helix model has been supported by studies applying glycosylation scanning, the use of epitope-tags placed within the extrafacial loops as well as antibodies directed against the predicted extra-and intracellular loops and the N-and C-terminal parts of the proteins. All family members are highly glycosylated membrane proteins harbouring an N-linked glycosylation site. For Class I and II family members this is positioned in the first exofacial loop between transmembrane helices 1 and 2, while class III family members contain a shorter extracellular loop 1 and harbor the glycosylation site within the larger loop 9 [3].

Sequence comparisons between all isoforms identified conserved residues that have been termed sugar transporter signatures [3]. These include conserved glycine residues in helices 1, 2, 4, 5, 7, 8 and 10, indicating a critical role in the structure of these helices. In particular helix 7 appears to be important for substrate binding from the exofacial site.

Nonetheless, the primary sequences of the various isoforms do not allow prediction of their substrate specificity or kinetics of transport. However, on the basis of mutational analyses, several residues and motifs have been demonstrated to participate in the substrate recognition by GLUT1 as well as other isoforms. GLUT1, 3, and 4, which transport glucose but not fructose, have the QLS sequence in helix 7.

GLUT2 and 5, which both transport fructose, have a HVA or MGG in this position. Structure function analysis of GLUT2 and 3 chimeras expressed in *Xenopus laevis* oocytes demonstrated that GLUT3 can be converted to a glucose/fructose transporter with GLUT2 transport kinetics when the amino acid sequence of GLUT2 from the beginning of helix 7 to the COOH terminus is inserted into GLUT3. This demonstrates the impact of helix7 on substrate specificity and kinetics of transport. A specific feature of all Class II transporters is their ability to transport fructose, with GLUT5 representing the *bona fide* fructose transporter. Again, helix7 is important for exofacial substrate recognition, since transport of fructose by class II isoforms has been linked to the presence of a NXV/NXI motif. Mutating the isoleucine position significantly reduced fructose transport, while glucose uptake was unaltered. Interestingly, Class II isoforms were unable to transport 2-deoxy-D-glucose (2-DG) or galactose. A valine to isoleucine mutation in GLUT2 (V165I) within helix 5 abolished 2-DG transport, and introduction of the same point mutation in GLUT1 also resulted in a comparable reduction of 2-DG transport.

For GLUT1, the topology and relative orientation of the 12 transmembrane helices with the outward-facing substrate-binding sites have been been proposed by two models. More than 50% of the complete polypeptide sequence has been analyzed by cysteine scanning mutagenesis using the substituted cysteine accessibility method (SCAM) allowing a detailed prediction of the exofacial substrate-binding site and the folding of the human GLUT1. A three-dimensional model for GLUT1 has been developed based on structural information from crystallized members of the major facilitator superfamily, glycerol-3-phosphate transporter and lactose permease. Binding of glucose, forskolin, and phloretin was predicted in close proximity to the exofacial vestibule in this model. While a second binding site for forskolin and phloretin was predicted at the intracellular portion of GLUT1, cytochalasin B has been docked only at one particular endofacial position of the protein.

4. Class I family members

Isoforms of Class I GLUTs are well characterized transporters with GLUT1 being the first isoform cloned and described in 1985.

4.1. GLUT1 (*Slc2a1*)

GLUT1, also known as the HepG2 or erythrocyte sugar transporter, is highly abundant in erythrocyte membranes making up 3-5% of the total erythrocyte proteins. The high amount of GLUT1 in red blood cells allowed the generation and characterization of an antibody that was used for the molecular cloning of GLUT1 from a hepatoma cDNA expression library in 1985 [26]. Although not present in hepatocytes, however, GLUT1 represents the most ubiquitously expressed isoform. The transporter is already found throughout early mammalian embryo development from the oocyte to the blastocyst and is present at high levels in endothelial and epithelial-like barriers of the brain, the eye, peripheral nerves, the placenta and especially in certain tumor cell lines and tissues, although not in hepatocytes. Also, GLUT1 is highly expressed in most routinely used laboratory cell lines.

When assessed in *Xenopus laevis* oocytes, GLUT1 transports glucose with a K_m of ~3 mM. Under equilibrium exchange conditions GLUT1 has a K_m of 20-21 mM for 3-O-methylglucose and 5 mM for 2-DG. Other hexoses transported by GLUT1 are galactose, mannose and glucosamine. When expressed in *S. cerevisae* rat GLUT1 showed a K_m for D-glucose of 3.4 mM and transport was inhibited by cytochalasin B (IC_{50}=0.44μM), $HgCl_2$ ($IC_5$0=3.5μM), phloretin (IC_{50}=49 μM) and phlorizin (IC_{50}=355 μM).

4.1.1. *GLUT1 physiology*

Human Physiology-the GLUT1 deficiency syndrome (OMIM #606777)

Mutations in the GLUT1 gene are causative for an autosomal-dominant disorder that is characterized by infantile seizures, developmental delay, acquired microcephaly, and ataxia and infantile seizures which is assumed to be caused by the decreased rate of glucose transport from the blood into cerebrospinal fluid. Defective glucose transport across the blood-brain barrier was first described 1991 [27] and linked to GLUT1 deficiency in 1998 [28]. About a 100 cases have been identified worldwide, including a wide spectrum of heterozygous mutations, including nonsense, missense, insertion, deletion and splice-site mutations, and hemizygosity of the GLUT1 gene.

Since ketone bodies bypass the blood-brain barrier and enter the brain via a monocarboxylic acid transporter (MCT1) they provide an alternative energy source for the brain under conditions of GLUT1 deficiency. Accordingly, a ketogenic diet is effective in controlling the seizures and other symptoms of the GLUT1 deficiency syndrome. However, this treatment is less effective regarding neurobehavioral symptoms. Correlations between genotype and phenotype still remain elusive.

Mouse Models of GLUT1 deficiency

Although representing the first GLUT isoform that was discovered, and despite being well characterized, mouse models for GLUT1 deficiency were only described recently. Mice that are transgenic for a homozygous GLUT1 anti-sense transgene are lethal during gestation; heterozygosity for the GLUT1 anti-sense cDNA was associated with growth retardation and developmental malformations.

In mice, homozygous knockout of GLUT1 was associated with embryonic lethality around day E10dpc and E13-14dpc, while heterozygous animals were viable and showed no differences in body weight development and growth. Decreased brain weights were reported, however, histological abnormalities were not found. While plasma glucose levels were normal in the heterozygous animals, glucose was decreased in the cerebrospinal fluid (CSF). As shown by PET-scan analysis, glucose uptake and metabolism were reduced in brains of heterozygous GLUT1 knockout animals. These animals also showed deficits in motor activity, balance and coordination as well as spontaneous cortical seizures. Overall, heterozygosity for GLUT1 in mice resembles features of humans with the GLUT1 deficiency syndrome.

4.2. GLUT2 *(Slc2a2)*

The second transporter of the GLUT family was cloned in 1988 from human liver and kidney cDNA libraries. The initial characterization detected GLUT2 mainly in the liver, kidney and intestine but the transporter was later demonstrated to be present specifically in the insulin producing β-cells of the pancreas. GLUT2 is a low-affinity, high capacity transporter and with a K_m in the range of ~17 mM, it has the highest K_m for glucose among the known members of the GLUT family. GLUT2 also transports galactose (~92 mM), D-mannose (~125 mM), and D-fructose (~76 mM). Recently, GLUT2 was shown to transport glucosamine with high affinity ($K_{m=}$~0.8 mM). Structurally, GLUT2 lacks the QLS motif in helix 7 which is thought to confer substrate specificity of the transporter, and which may explain the high affinity for glucosamine.

GLUT2 is located in the basolateral membrane of the epithelial cells of the intestine and kidney, where it participates in the release of absorbed (via SGLT1 in the intestine) or reabsorbed (via SGLT1 and 2 in the kidney) glucose into the blood stream.

4.2.1. GLUT2 physiology

Human GLUT2 deficiency and the FANCONI-BICKEL SYNDROME (OMIM #227810)

Rare homozygous or compound heterozygous mutations within the GLUT2 gene cause a type of glycogen storage diseases (GSD), termed GSD XI. The first patient was described by Fanconi and Bickel's, therefore the GLUT2 deficiency is referred to as Fanconi-Bickel Syndrome (FBS). Thus far, 112 patients have been reported. Analysis of 63 patients revealed a total of 34 different *GLUT2* mutations with none of them being particularly frequent. The clinical symptoms of FBS are hepatomegaly secondary to glycogen accumulation, glucose and galactose intolerance, fasting hypoglycemia, tubular nephropathy, and severely stunted growth. In contrast to the metabolism of glucose and galactose, utilization of orally or intravenously administered fructose is normal in FBS patients.

Glucose homeostasis in FBS-patients is heavily disturbed and postprandial hyperglycemia is frequently observed. A few patients have been diagnosed with diabetes mellitus and have been treated with insulin. Hypoglycemia in fasting states is a feature of FBS. Hypoglycemia has very frequently been documented and plasma glucose levels as low as 18 mg/dl have been reported in FBS patients. Compared to other types of hepatic glycogen diseases hepatic adenomas or malignancies have never been observed in patients with FBS.

No specific treatment exists for patients with FBS. Symptomatic treatment is directed towards stabilization of glucose homeostasis and compensation for renal losses of various solutes. The amelioration of the consequences of renal tubulopathy includes the replacement of water and electrolytes. In order to control renal glucose loss and hepatic glycogen accumulation in FBS, patients receive a diet with adequate caloric intake with slowly absorbed carbohydrates.

The importance of GLUT2 in the regulation of glucose-stimulated insulin secretion from the β-cell of the islets of Langerhans has been well established for mice.

Investigations of GLUT2 mutations that have been linked to the Fanconi-Bickel syndrome [29] or patients with transient or permanent neonatal diabetes mellitus [30] indicated an important role for this transporter in pancreatic β-cell development and function in humans.

Mouse models of GLUT2 deficiency

The consequences of GLUT2 deficiency have been analyzed in detail for the various tissues where GLUT2 is involved and/or essential in maintaining whole body glucose homeostasis. Early on, the critical role for GLUT2 in the β-cell for glucose stimulated insulin-secretion *in vivo* became apparent in mice with transgenic overexpression of a GLUT2 antisense RNA specifically in pancreatic β-cell cells. Upon an 80% reduction of GLUT2 in β-cells those animals display hyperglycemia and develop diabetes.

Whole body GLUT2 knockout in mice results in offspring that appears completely normal at birth, but neonates develop early symptoms similar to type 2 diabetes and do not survive beyond the age of 3 weeks. Homozygous GLUT2 deficiency in mice results in hyperglycemia and elevated plasma levels of free fatty acids and β-hydroxybutyrate. *In vivo* glucose tolerance is abnormal and, *in vitro*, β-cells display a gradual loss of control of insulin gene expression by glucose. Glucose stimulated insulin secretion in islets was impaired by loss of the first, but not the second phase of insulin secretion. GLUT2 knockout mice show marked hyperglucagonemia, and this is accompanied by alterations in the postnatal development of pancreatic islets, evidenced by a gradual inversion of the α-to β-cell ratio. A direct link between diet induced insulin resistance and β-cell dysfunction via disturbed GLUT2 plasma membrane localization has recently been demonstrated. Administration of a high-fat diet feeding in mice results in intracellular retention of the transporter due to improper glycosylation of the protein thereby leading to compromised glucose stimulated insulin secretion.

The early lethality of GLUT2 deficient mice shortly after birth hindered the analysis of GLUT2 physiology in the different tissues of its expression. Transgenic mice that overexpress GLUT1 specifically in β-cells under the control of the rat insulin promoter were generated (RIPGLUT1/GLUT2$^{-/-}$) to study the functional consequences of GLUT2 deficiency in tissues such as liver, kidney, intestine, and also in the brain.

In the liver, GLUT2 deficiency was expected to dramatically affect hepatic glucose output under fasting conditions. Interestingly, hepatic glucose output and glucagon response of the livers from mice lacking GLUT2 were normal. No counterregulation of other transporters known at that time was observed (GLUT1, 3, 4, 5 and SGLT1). Glucose output in GLUT2 deficient livers was not inhibited by cytochalasin B. An alternative membrane traffic-based pathway was proposed that releases glucose directly from the ER after glycogen breakdown or gluconeogenesis. The exact nature of this route has not been determined. In humans GLUT2 deficiency is associated with a marked hypoglycemia in the fasting state owing to a diminished hepatic glucose output and a failure of glucagon to increase plasma glucose. However, human patients with FBS do not generally develop diabetes and do not display a complete loss of their beta cell function, indicating that functionality of human pancreatic β-cells does not solely depend on GLUT2.

Deletion of GLUT2 specifically in the liver [31] or the central nervous system [32] showed, that GLUT2 mediated glucose-sensing mechanisms in both organs exist which control pancreatic β cell mass and function.

In the kidney, a role for GLUT2 in basolateral sugar reabsorption by tubular epithelial cells was postulated due the glucosuria that has been observed in RIPGLUT1/GLUT2$^{-/-}$mice. GLUT2 complements the active sugar uptake at the apical epithelium mediated by SGLT2. The functional relevance for GLUT2 in the kidney in humans is supported by the observation of impaired kidney glucose reabsorption in patients with FBS.

4.3. GLUT3 *(SLC2A3)*

GLUT3 was cloned from a human fetal muscle cDNA library. GLUT3 is considered as a neuron-specific glucose transporter due to its dominant expression in the brain in various species. However, besides the brain GLUT3 is also expressed in tissues with high demand for glucose such as testes (spermatozoa), placenta, preimplantation embryos or certain cancer cells and cancer tissues. Its tissue distribution and function correspond with its high affinity (K_m=1.4 mM for 2-DG), and transport capacity for glucose. While galactose (K_m=8.5 mM), mannose,

http://dx.doi.org/10.5772/58325

maltose, xylose and dehydroascorbic acid are substrates for GLUT3, fructose is not. GLUT3 is inhibited by cytochalasin B (Ki=0.4 μM), phloretin, and and phlorizin.

4.3.1. GLUT3 physiology

Single nucleotide polymorphisms (SNP's) in the GLUT3 gene have been identified and linked to dyslexia

Dyslexia is one of the most common learning disorders in school-aged children. Dyslexic children show differences in event-related potential measurements, in particular for mismatch negativity (MMN), which reflects automatic speech deviance processing. Whole-genome association analysis in 200 dyslexic children, focusing on MMN measurements, identified two SNPs that both showed a significant association with mRNA-expression levels of *SLC2A3* on chromosome 12. It was suggested that a possible trans-regulation effect on *SLC2A3* might lead to glucose deficits in dyslexic children that might cause their attenuated MMN in passive listening tasks.

Mouse Models of GLUT3 deficiency

During mouse preimplantation development GLUT3 is expressed at the apical membrane of the trophectoderm layer of the blastocyst and mediates glucose uptake by the embryo from the external (maternal) environment. Knockdown of the transporter by antisense-RNA at this time-point of development disrupts blastocyst development by diminishing uptake of glucose by the embryo. These data indicated a crucial role for GLUT3 during preimplantation embryo development and its deficiency in mice was assumed to result in embryonic lethality before implantation. Indeed, homozygous loss of GLUT3 leads to a complete loss of embryos at day 12.5. However, morulae develop normally to the blastocyst stage and implantation is not affected by loss of GLUT3.

Heterozygous GLUT3 knockout mice have been characterized especially for a potential neuron (brain) specific phenotype. These animals exhibit significantly enhanced cerebrocortical activity and are slightly more sensitive to an acoustic startle stimulus. However, behavior of these animals regarding coordination, reflexes, motor abilities, anxiety, learning, and memory is normal.

Zhao et al. described features of autism spectrum disorders in heterozygous GLUT3 knockout animals as being abnormal spatial learning, working memory, electroencephalographic seizures, and perturbed social behavior with reduced vocalization and stereotypes at low frequency.

4.4. GLUT4 *(SLC2A4)*

Besides GLUT1, GLUT4 represents one of the most intensively studied glucose transporters which is attributed to its important physiological role regulating the rate-limiting step in insulin-stimulated glucose uptake of skeletal and cardiac muscle, brown and white adipose tissue. Thereby, impaired GLUT4 translocation is causally linked to insulin resistance and consequently to the disease condition of non-insulin dependent diabetes mellitus.

GLUT4 was cloned in 1989 by various groups from human, rat, and mouse tissues. GLUT4 displays a similar affinity for glucose as GLUT1 with a K_m of ~5 mM, and is also capable of transporting dehydroascorbic acid and glucosamine (K_m ~3.9 mM). When expressed in yeast (*S. cerevisae*) rat GLUT4 is inhibited by the classical inhibitors cytochalasin B (IC50=0.2 μM), phloretin (IC50=10 μM) and phlorizin (IC50=140 μM).

4.5. GLUT4 signalling and cell biology

GLUT4 contains unique sorting motifs at its N-terminus (FQQI) and C-terminus (dileucine) are critical for its capability to traffic between specific intracellular compartments and translocate to the plasma membrane in response to different stimuli. Insulin and exercise are able to rapidly and acutely stimulate GLUT4 translocation to the plasma membrane and thereby influence glucose uptake in muscle and adipose tissue via distinct signalling mechanisms. Activation of the insulin receptor (IR) leads to its autophosphorylation and subsequent signalling through the insulin receptor substrate proteins (IRS) and recruitment of PI 3-kinase catalyzes the formation of phosphatidylinositol (3,4,5)-3-phosphate (PIP3). PIP3 itself activates the protein kinase Akt via two intermediate protein kinases, PDK1 and Rictor/ mTOR. Akt2 rather than the Akt1 or Akt3 isoforms appears to control GLUT4 trafficking. With the identification of the Akt substrates TBC1D4 (AS160), and more recently TBC1D1, two GTPase activating proteins have been identified that appear to bridge the gap between insulin-signalling and trafficking events. For TBC1D4 the substrate is the rab GTPase rab10 which has been shown to be required for insulin-stimulated translocation of GLUT4 vesicles to the plasma membrane.

Exercise has also been shown to induce TBC1D4 phosphorylation but apparently via a distinct PI3-kinase independent mechanism that requires activation of AMPK. However, simultaneous disruption of AMPK and Akt failed to completely inhibit contraction-induced AS160 phosphorylation hinting towards alternative signalling events leading to GLUT4 translocation. A PI 3-kinase-independent pathway has been proposed that involves the adaptor molecules APS and CAP that bind to the insulin receptor and recruit c-Cbl. C-Cbl signals to the guanine nucleotide exchange factor C3G which activates the small GTP binding protein TC10. However, recent data indicated a rather minor contribution for this pathway in insulin mediated GLUT4 translocation.

4.5.1. GLUT4 physiology

Human

Although the significance of GLUT4 for insulin-stimulated glucose uptake in muscle and adipose tissue is well understood, thus far, no polymorphisms within the GLUT4 gene have been identified that would robustly be associated with impaired glucose homeostasis in humans under circumstances such as type 2 diabetes, increased fasting blood glucose levels, or obesity.

Mouse Models of GLUT4 deficiency

Conventional Knockout

GLUT4 knockout mice, surprisingly, are normoglycemic with insulin resistance and hyperinsulinemia in the fed state. The mice are growth-retarded, with markedly reduced fat mass, cardiomegaly, and shortened lifespan, but no diabetes. In contrast, heterozygous GLUT4-null mice develop hyperglycemia and hyperinsulinemia associated with reduced muscle glucose uptake, hypertension and morphological alterations in heart and liver. Rather unexpectedly, about 50% of heterozygous GLUT4 knockout mice develop diabetes before the age of 6 months, a phenotype that can be reversed by selective overexpression of GLUT4 in skeletal muscle.

Muscle-specific GLUT4 knockout mice

In contrast to conventional GLUT4 knockout animals muscle specific GLUT4 deficient mice have normal body and fat pad weight and a normal lifespan. While skeletal muscle mass is unchanged the heart weight is increased similar to GLUT4 deficient mice and heart specific GLUT4 knockout animals. Basal and especially insulin-or contraction-induced glucose uptake into skeletal muscle is reduced, which is causative for the hyperglycemia, glucose intolerance and insulin resistance seen in those animals. A subset of animals develops diabetes. Surprisingly, insulin stimulated glucose transport in adipose tissue and insulin induced suppression of hepatic glucose production are also impaired which is assumed to be secondary to the hyperglycemia in those animals.

Adipose tissue-specific GLUT4 knockout mice

Adipose tissue selective GLUT4 inactivation, unlike the conventional GLUT4 disruption, does not affect growth, adipose mass or size. Cardiac hypertrophy is not seen in those animals. Fat specific GLUT4 null mice are insulin resistant and glucose intolerant and a subset of animals develop diabetes, which is also observed in muscle specific GLUT4 deficient mice. Muscle and liver are insulin-resistant in those animals. Surprisingly, insulin resistance in muscle was only observed in vivo but not ex vivo indicating a systemic impact of adipose tissue on insulin sensitivity.

Cardiac tissue specific GLUT4 knockout mice

GLUT4 knockout mice specifically muscle and cardiac tissue specific GLUT4 deficient mice all develop cardiac hypertrophy. While homo-and heterozygous GLUT4 null mice show cardiac dysfunction under normal conditions, cardiac specific GLUT4 knockouts have normal contractile function under basal conditions but decreased recovery after hypoxia. Metabolically, heart specific GLUT4 knockout mice are normal and have a normal lifespan.

4.6. GLUT14 *(SLC2A14)*

Searching the human genome for additional genes coding for glucose transporters, a putative gene was identified and cloned showing 95% identity to GLUT3 on the nucleotide level. The *SLC2A14* gene maps to chromosome 12p13.3 with a 10Mb distance to GLUT3 and appears to be a consequence of a gene duplication of GLUT3. GLUT14 was shown to be specifically expressed in the testes. Two alternatively spliced forms of GLUT14 were identified. Interestingly, GLUT14 has no orthologue in mice, a finding that has also been made for GLUT11.

4.7. Class II family members

With GLUT5 being identified in 1990 and established as a fructose transporter initial transport studies for GLUT7 and 9 indicated that those transporters might also transport fructose. A specific feature for class II transporters is that cytochalasin B as a classical GLUT inhibitor does not block glucose transport. Furthermore, all isoforms do not show an affinity for 2-DG and galactose. Unique for GLUT9 and GLUT11 is the alternative splicing /promoter usage, where either two or three different mRNA's are transcribed, respectively. In case of GLUT9 this leads to two proteins that only differ in their N-terminal region.

4.8. GLUT5 *(SLC2A5)*

Human GLUT5 was initially cloned from an intestinal epithelial cell line. GLUT5 is considered as the prototypic fructose transporter – when expressed in *Xenopus laevis* oocytes the human protein transports fructose with a K_m of 6 mM without any noticeable glucose transport activity. However, fructose transport is not inhibited by cytochalasin B, phloretin or phlorizin. Besides fructose, the rat GLUT5 transports glucose, an activity that can be blocked by cytochalasin B. In humans, rats and mice, GLUT5 is primarily expressed in the jejunal region of the small intestine. Lower levels of the protein are expressed in the kidney, the brain, skeletal muscle, and adipose tissue. GLUT5 mediates fructose absorption in the jejunum at the apical, and potentially, at the basolateral membrane, of the epithelial cells into the portal vein (Figure 3B).

4.8.1. GLUT5 physiology

Mouse Models of GLUT5 deficiency

GLUT5 deficiency is associated with reduced fructose absorption when animals are challenged by a high fructose diet. While wildtype mice upon high fructose feeding display an enhanced salt absorption in their jejuna and develop systemic hypertension, GLUT5 knockout mice do not show fructose stimulated salt absorption. Instead, the animals display impaired nutrient absorption that is accompanied by hypotension. Absence of GLUT5 leads to a massive dilatation of the cecum and colon, consistent with severe malabsorption. On a normal chow diet, GLUT5 deficient mice have normal blood pressure and display normal weight gain. The phenotype of GLUT5 deficient mice demonstrates that this isoform is essential for fructose absorption by the intestine and thereby fundamentally involved in fructose induced hypertension.

4.9. GLUT7 *(SLC2A7)*

The human GLUT7 was cloned from an intestinal cDNA library using a PCR-based strategy. GLUT7 is primarily expressed in the small intestine and colon, although mRNA has been detected in the testes and prostate as well. The protein has been localized to the apical membrane of the small intestine and colon. GLUT7 shows a rather high affinity for glucose and fructose (K_m for glucose=0.3mM) while galactose, 2-DG, and xylose are not transported. Sugar transport by GLUT7 is not inhibited by cytochalasin B or phloretin. Sequence alignments between fructose and non-fructose transporting GLUT isoforms identified a motif in GLUT7 that potentially confers its ability to transport fructose. Mutational analysis of those residues in GLUT7 identified isoleucine 314 as an important determinant for fructose affinity. The finding of a specific residue within the extracellular vestibule of helix 7 that drives substrate specificity was extended to GLUT2, 5, 9 and 11 and proposed as a common NXI/V consensus motif among isoforms capable of transporting fructose.

4.10. GLUT9 *(SLC2A9)*

Human GLUT9 cDNA was isolated by PCR amplification from a human kidney cDNA library on the basis of sequence information from ESTs and from its genomic sequence. GLUT9 mRNA is detected almost exclusively in the kidney and liver and at low levels in the small intestine, placenta, lung and leucocytes. GLUT9 is localized to the insulin-secreting β-cells of human and mouse islets, where downregulation of the protein by siRNA in rat and mouse insulinoma cells leads to a reduced glucose-stimulated insulin secretion. In humans as well as in mice alternative splicing/or promoter usage results in two proteins, GLUT9a and GLUT9b, which only differ in their N-terminal region. While human and mouse GLUT9b are mainly expressed in the kidney, placenta and liver, GLUT9a shows a broader tissue distribution. The different N-termini of human GLUT9a and b determine basolateral versus apical sorting in polarized cells *in vitro*, respectively. In mouse kidney, GLUT9 is localized to apical as well as basolateral membranes of distal convoluted tubules. Initial characterization of GLUT9 determined a rather low affinity for 2-DG. However, a high affinity transport has been reported for glucose and fructose with K_m values of 0.6 mM and 0.4 mM, respectively. More recently, GLUT9 has been identified as a high-affinity uric acid transporter with a K_m of 0.9 mM and 0.6 mM for the human and mouse protein, respectively. Although transport of glucose and fructose has not been observed by some investigators, GLUT9 is thought to exchange glucose or fructose for urate. The classical inhibitor cytochalasin B does not block GLUT9 function. GLUT9 has been established to represent a major regulator of urate homeostasis in dogs, mice, and men.

4.10.1. GLUT9 physiology

In humans GLUT9 is involved in renal uric acid reabsorption-mutations in the GLUT9 gene have consequences on plasma uric acid levels

Various genome wide association studies uncovered polymorphisms in *SLC2A9* as being one of the most significantly associated genes that can be linked to gout and increased serum uric acid concentrations. Although the identified SNPs are located in intronic regions of the gene, evidence exists that increased RNA expression for GLUT9 positively correlates with increased serum uric acid concentrations. In contrast, exonic mutations in GLUT9 suggested that loss of GLUT9 function is associated with hypouricemia. Two distinct heterozygous missense mutations (R380W and R198C in GLUT9a) were described in three patients with hypouricemia. The two mutations were shown to result in loss of function when uric acid transport was studied in *Xenopus laevis* oocyes. A genome-wide homozygosity screen linked hereditary hypouricemia to two homozygous SLC2A9 mutations that lead to a missense mutation (L75R) or a 36-kb deletion. The homozygous loss-of-function mutations of GLUT9 caused a total defect of uric acid absorption, leading to severe hypouricemia complicated by nephrolithiasis and exercise-induced acute renal failure. Therefore, GLUT9 is essential for renal reabsorption of uric acid-increased expression is associated with hyperuricemia and gout, while loss of function leads to severe hypouricemia.

Mouse Models of GLUT9 deficiency

GLUT9 deficiency in mice leads to hyperuricemia, massive hyperuricosuria, and an early-onset nephropathy, which his is in contrast to the condition in humans where dysfunctional GLUT9 is associated with hypouricemia. Hyperuricemia in mice due to GLUT9 deficiency appears to be a result of impaired urid acid uptake by the liver and therefore inability to be degraded to allantoin by uricase. The nephropathy in GLUT9 knockout animals is characterized by obstructive lithiasis, tubulointerstitial inflammation, and progressive inflammatory fibrosis of the cortex. In contrast, liver-specific GLUT9 inactivation in adult mice results in severe hyperuricemia and hyperuricosuria, in the absence of urate nephropathy or any structural abnormality of the kidney. The deficiency of GLUT9 in mice showed that it represents a functional uric acid transporter *in vivo,* allowing GLUT9 to be identified as a major player in urate homeostasis due to its dual role in uric acid handling in the kidney and in the liver. Whether GLUT9 at all plays a role as a (glucose)/fructose transporter that potentially links fructose uptake by the liver and uric acid metabolism remains to be seen (Figure 4A).

4.11. GLUT11 *(SLC2A11)*

The human GLUT11 was cloned by PCR on the basis of sequence information obtained from ESTs and a genomic sequence. Three variants of GLUT11 (GLUT11-A, GLUT11-B, and GLUT11-C) have been identified that only differ in their N-terminal sequences. Since for each of the variants the corresponding 5′ sequences upstream of exon 1 exhibit promoter activity, transcriptional regulation is assumed to occur by alternative promoter usage. The three isoforms are expressed in a tissue specific manner: GLUT11-A is present in heart, skeletal muscle and kidney; GLUT11-B is expressed in placental, adipose, and kidney tissue; while GLUT11-C is found in adipose, heart, skeletal muscle and pancreatic tissue. Glucose transport activity for GLUT11 was detected in liposomes reconstituted with GLUT11 containing membranes. The transporter shows affinity for glucose with a K_m of 0.16 mM when measured in *Xenopus laevis* oocytes. GLUT11 also transports fructose but not galactose and shows a rather low affinity for cytochalasin B. Mutational analysis of the DSV motif in GLUT11 that corresponds to the "fructose" transporter motif "NAI" also showed that also in GLUT11 this particular region of helix 7 determines substrate selectivity of the transporter. Endogenous GLUT11 protein was localized in heart and skeletal muscle tissue with an antibody raised against the C-terminus of GLUT11 that does not distinguish between the different variants. Human GLUT11 is expressed exclusively in slow-twitch muscle fibres and is unaffected by physiological and pathophysiological conditions except in primary myopathy. Surprisingly, the human SLC2A11 gene has not orthologue in the rat and mouse genome.

4.12. Class III family members

Class III isoforms share specific features that are unique to this Class. First, structurally all Class III members carry their N-glycosylation site at the fifth extracellular loop. Common to all the isoforms is the presence of an internalization signal (dileucine or YSRI in case of GLUT10) that retains these transporters at an intracellular localization under steady state conditions. Thus far, a stimulus for translocation of Class III isoforms leading to plasma membrane localization has only been proposed for GLUT13 which has not been confirmed.

4.13. GLUT6 *(SLC2A6)*

GLUT6 (formerly designated GLUT9) was cloned from human leucoyte cDNA by (RACE)-PCR on the basis of murine ESTs and the human genomic sequence. GLUT6 mRNA is expressed predominantly in the brain, spleen and peripheral leucocytes. Hexose transport for GLUT6 was only shown when reconstituted in liposomes, where GLUT6 transport activity was found in the presence of 5 mM but not 1 mM glucose. GLUT6 exhibits a low cytochalasin B binding affinity. Thus far, no other data on kinetics of transport and potential substrates have been published for this isoform.

GLUT6 contains an N-terminal dileucine motif that is responsible for intracellular retention of the protein when overexpressed in primary rat adipocytes. GLUT6 is only detected at the plasma membrane when the dileucine residues are mutated to alanine or when clathrin dependent endocytosis is blocked by overexpression of a dominant-negative dynamin mutant. However, no cell-surface translocation of GLUT6 is observed in response to stimuli such as insulin, phorbol ester or hyperosmolarity. A gene expression profiling study aimed to identify deregulated in chronic lymphocytic leukaemia associated with Trisomy 12 identified Slc2a6 among the seven genes with the strongest correlation. Although a significant deregulation was not confirmed subsequently by real-time PCR analysis, the specific expression of GLUT6 in leucocytes and the spleen might indicate an important role for this transporter in normal physiology for this cell lineage.

The biochemistry, cell biology and physiology of GLUT6 is currently not well understood.

4.14. GLUT8 *(SLC2A8)*

GLUT8 (formerly GLUTX1) was the first isoform of the extended *SLC2A* family to be identified by database mining. The human, rat and mouse cDNA were cloned by 5′ and 3′ RACE-PCR from testis cDNA samples. The transporter is mainly expressed in the testes, and lower levels are found in the brain (cerebellum), adrenal gland, liver, spleen, brown adipose tissue and lung. Functional characterization of GLUT8 in *Xenopus laevis* oocytes immediately revealed the intracellular retention of the transporter due to the presence of a dileucine based motif in its N-terminus. When the two leucine residues are changed to alanines GLUT8 localizes to the plasma membrane in mammalian cells and *Xenopus laevis* oocytes that allowed the determination of transport kinetics for the protein. GLUT8 shows a high affinity for glucose with a K_m of ~2 mM. Glucose transport can be competitively inhibited with fructose, galactose, and cytochalasin B. The intracellular localization of

GLUT8 raised the question of whether this isoform would be insulin-responsive and thereby compensate for GLUT4 in the respective knockout mice which are lacking the insulin-responsive glucose transporter yet near normal glucose tolerance. Indeed, in blastocysts of mice, GLUT8 has been found to account for insulin-stimulated glucose uptake. However, various groups performed extensive studies in primary rat adipocytes, 3T3L1 adipocytes, insulin-responsive CHO-cells as well as neuronal cell types such as N2A, PC12, and hippocampal neurons that all failed to identify a stimulus that leads to a plasma membrane translocation of GLUT8.

The intracellular localization of GLUT8 is also observed *in vivo* under steady-state conditions. In the testis immunofluorescence microscopy shows intracellular localization of GLUT8 in a late-endosomal/lysosomal compartment. In the brain, immunogold labeling electron-microscopy localized GLUT8 in synaptic dense core vesicles of nerve terminals and secretory granules of vasopressin neurons.

The intracellular retention signal of GLUT8 has been characterized and found to contain the consensus sequence [D/E]XXXL[L/I] that represents a late-endosomal/lysosomal sorting motif. The DEXXXLL sorting signal of GLUT8 interacts with the adaptor proteins AP-1 and AP-2 and controls trafficking of the protein. Interestingly, both GLUT8 and GLUT12 contain a [D/E]XXXL[L/I] sorting signal; however, the exact composition of the XXX residues seems to fine-tune the routing and trafficking of the two proteins.

4.14.1. GLUT8 physiology

Mouse Models of GLUT8 deficiency

GLUT8 knockout mice appear healthy and exhibit normal growth, body weight development and glycemic control, indicating that GLUT8 does not play a significant role in maintenance of whole body glucose homeostasis. Offspring distribution from heterozygous matings indicated a deviation from the expected Mendelian distribution regarding birth of GLUT8 homozygous animals. This observation was attributed to a decreased sperm motility of GLUT8 deficient spermatocytes that is associated with lower ATP levels and a reduced mitochondrial membrane potential, while number and survival rate of spermatozoa is unchanged. The reduced amount of homozygous GLUT8 offspring is not related to impaired preimplantation embryo development – as might have been suggested by antisense studies in embryos-since mating of knockout mice produced viable, normally developing offspring in numbers comparable to those of a wildtype intercross. GLUT8 deficiency is associated with behavioural alterations indicating a significant physiological role for this isoform in the central nervous system. GLUT8 deficient mice have an increased proliferation of hippocampal cells and behavioral tests show increased arousal, a tendency to altered grooming, and a reduced risk assessment in those animals. However, despite the in depth characterization of the cell biology of GLUT8 and its physiology *in vivo* based on knockout mice, the function of the protein remains thus far unknown.

4.15. GLUT10 *(SLC2A10)*

GLUT10 has been cloned from human liver cDNA by 3′ and 5′ RACE PCR based on an EST sequence that was identified via a homology search with known GLUT protein sequences. GLUT10 mRNA is present in the human heart, lung, brain, liver, skeletal muscle, pancreas, placenta and kidney. Expression of GLUT10 is also detected in human and mouse white adipose tissue as well as human and mouse adipocyte cell lines SGBS and 3T3L1, respectively. One remarkable structural feature is the absence of the PESPR motif just after helix 6 that is conserved for all the GLUT isoforms. Heterologous expression of GLUT10 in *Xenopus laevis* oocytes demonstrated 2-DG transport with high affinity (K_m ~0.3 mM). Uptake of 2-DG can be competed with galactose and glucose and inhibited with phloretin.

Although no localization study has been performed for GLUT10 clearly demonstrating a plasma membrane or intracellular localization as seen for other Class III family members, immunocytochemical studies indicated an intracellular localization for GLUT10 under steady-state conditions. The presence of the potential internalization motif YSRI at the C terminus of the transporter supports these findings.

GLUT10 is located at the chromosomal region 20q12-13.1, a susceptibility locus that has been linked to type 2 diabetes in Caucasian Americans. Therefore, there has been particular interest in GLUT10 as a potential candidate or susceptibility gene involved in the disease. However, polymorphisms in GLUT10 were not associated to type 2 diabetes in Caucasian Americans, Danish, Finns, and Taiwanese populations.

4.15.1. GLUT10 physiology

GLUT10 and Arterial tortuosity syndrome (ATS, OMIM# 208050) in Humans

Deficiency for GLUT10 in humans has been found to be associated with ATS, a rare autosomal recessive connective tissue disease that is characterized by widespread arterial involvement with elongation, tortuosity, and aneurysms of the arteries. Homozygous mutations (deletion, non-sense, and missense) for GLUT10 were found in six families with ATS. It is currently unknown how loss of GLUT10 leads to this connective tissue disorder [33].

Mouse models of GLUT10 deficiency

Two groups reported the phenotypic analysis of mice with amino acid substitutions G128E or S150F in GLUT10 [34, 35]. Both substitutions are located in exon2 of GLUT10 and are conserved among the rodent and human protein. Based on predictions, the substitutions G128E and S150F were expected to interfere with the helix structure of transmembrane regions 4 and 5, respectively. The mice strains were generated after screening a mutant mouse library that was based on N-ethyl-N-nitrosurea (ENU) mutagenesis in healthy C3HeB/FeJ males. Callewaert et al. [34] did not report any of the vascular, anatomical, or immunohistological abnormalities as encountered in patients with ATS. Both mutant strains appear normal at birth, gained weight appropriately and survived to adulthood. The animals showed normal heart rhythm, heart structure, and ventricular function. No specific arterial tortuosity, stenosis, dilatation, or aneurysm in cerebral vessel pattern was noted. However, histopathology revealed thickening and an irregular vessel wall shape of arteries with increased elastic fibers. Furthermore, the animals displayed endothelial hypertrophy and disarranged elastic fibers that resulted in disruption of internal elastic lamina in the aorta. Neither group analyzed whether the mutations caused any dysfunction or loss of the target protein, therefore the reported phenotype of those mice remains inconclusive with respect to GLUT10 function.

4.16. GLUT12 *(SLC2A12)*

GLUT12 was identified by 5′ and 3′ RACE-PCR from the human breast cancer cell line MCF-7. Strong GLUT12 expression is found in ductal cell carcinoma *in situ* when compared to benign ducts of breast cancer tissues. GLUT12 is mainly expressed in skeletal muscle, heart, small intestine, adipose tissue, and prostate. GLUT12 shows glucose transport when functionally characterized in *Xenopus laevis* oocytes that can be competed with fructose, galactose, 2-DG, and cytochalasin B. The transport activity of GLUT12 has been demonstrated to be affected by pH and in other reports by sodium, indicating its activity might be directly or indirectly coupled to an electrochemical gradient.

As a Class III isoform GLUT12 also contains a dileucine motif – both at the N-and C-terminal ends of the protein. Furthermore, the transporter does not contain GLUT12 contains a hydrophobic residue in position 314 which has been implicated in case of the isoleucine for GLUT2, 5, and 7 with the capability of fructose transport. This structural feature goes along with the substrate specificity of GLUT1. Endogenous as well as overexpressed GLUT12 protein localizes to intracellular compartments as well as to the plasma membrane in various cell lines. The N-terminal dileucine signal of GLUT12 is similar to that of GLUT8 which is the [DE]XXXL[LI] consensus sequence that represents a late endosomal/lysosomal sorting signal. However, GLUT12 does not colocalize with GLUT8, but rather resides in the Golgi network and at the plasma membrane. Plasma membrane associated GLUT12 is not endocytosed, which indicates the absence of a continuous cycling mechanism for GLUT12.

The phenotypic characterization of mice deficient in GLUT4 indicates the presence of a second transporter that facilitates insulin-stimulated glucose transport. Due to its tissue expression and its biological characteristics, GLUT12 was studied for its ability to respond to insulin-induced plasma membrane translocation of the protein. Indeed, in human skeletal muscle insulin induces an increase in plasma membrane GLUT12 which is comparable to the insulin-stimulated GLUT4 translocation. Although GLUT12 expression in skeletal muscle is unaltered under pathophysiological conditions such as of obesity and type 2 diabetes these data imply that an additional transporter is expressed in human muscle that is insulin-responsive in a PI3-kinase dependent manner. Mice with transgenic overexpression of GLUT12 display increased insulin sensitivity in insulin-sensitive tissues, while basal (non-stimulated) glucose uptake into adipose tissue and skeletal muscle was unaffected [36] indicating that GLUT12 might contribute to insulin-stimulated glucose uptake in those tissues, an effect not observed in heart muscle. Besides its potential importance for substrate transport in insulin-sensitive tissues, GLUT12 also appears relevant in prostate and breast cancer. However, the physiological role and relevance for GLUT12 remains elusive [37].

4.17. GLUT13; HMIT *(SLC2A13)*

Screening of public expressed sequence databases with the GLUT8 protein sequence identified a rat EST clone that allowed cloning of the rat and human HMIT (*SLC2A13*) cDNAs from spleen and frontal cortex cDNA libraries. Despite low level expression in adipose tissue and kidney, HMIT is predominantly expressed in the brain, with high expression found in hippocampus, hypothalamus, cerebellum and brainstem.

The HMIT amino acid sequence contains all motifs known to be important for glucose transport activity. As for other Class III GLUT family members, HMIT is restricted to an intracellular location. Functional characterization of the protein in *Xenopus laevis* oocytes and in mammalian cells has been possible through the introduction of various mutations that yielded significant plasma membrane expression. Surprisingly, no sugar transport activity has been found for HMIT. Instead, HMIT has been identified as a H^+-coupled myoinositol symporter with a K_m of about 100 μM. More recently, HMIT has been shown to transport inositol-3-phosphate (IP3). HMIT is inhibited by the common GLUT inhibitors phloretin, phlorizin and cytochalasin B, although at high concentrations. Translocation of HMIT to the plasma membrane has been demonstrated to occur in PC12 cells or primary neurons upon depolarization or protein kinase C (PKC) activation resulting in functional HMIT at the plasma membrane evidenced by increased myoinositol uptake in those cells. However, those initial findings were not reproduced by other groups leaving uncertainty about a stimulus that induces plasma membrane translocation of the transporter. In the brain, myo-inositol serves as the precursor for phosphatidylinositol, a key regulator for various signaling pathways. Dysregulation of the phosphatidylinositol signaling has been implicated in psychiatric illness such as bipolar disorder. Standard therapies (lithium, valproic acid and carbamazepine) alter neuronal growth cone morphology, a phenotype that is reversed by extracellular myo-inositol. Because of its predominant expression in the brain compared to two other myo-inositol transporters that are sodium-coupled (SMIT1 and SMIT2), interest has been raised as to whether HMIT might play a role in the regulation of myo-inositol/phosphatidylinositol physiology in neurons. Mice deficient for the transporter demonstrated that HMIT is not involved in the neuronal transport of inositol from the extracellular environment.

Author details

Robert Augustin* and Eric Mayoux

*Address all correspondence to: Robert.Augustin@boehringer-ingelheim.com

Department of Cardiometabolic Diseases Research, Boehringer-Ingelheim Pharma GmbH&Co KG, Germany

References

[1] Wright EM, Loo DD, Hirayama BA. Biology of human sodium glucose transporters. Physiol Rev. 2011 Apr;91(2):733-94.

[2] Uldry M, Thorens B. The SLC2 family of facilitated hexose and polyol transporters. Pflugers Arch. 2004 Feb;447(5):480-9.

[3] Joost HG, Thorens B. The extended GLUT-family of sugar/polyol transport facilitators: nomenclature, sequence characteristics, and potential function of its novel members (review). Mol Membr Biol. 2001 Oct-Dec;18(4):247-56.

[4] Augustin R. The protein family of glucose transport facilitators: It's not only about glucose after all. IUBMB Life. 2010 May;62(5):315-33.

[5] Crane RK. Intestinal absorption of sugars. Physiol Rev. 1960 Oct;40:789-825.

[6] Ehrenkranz JR, Lewis NG, Kahn CR, Roth J. Phlorizin: a review. Diabetes Metab Res Rev. 2005 Jan-Feb;21(1):31-8.

[7] Lindquist B, Meeuwisse GW. Chronic diarrhoea caused by monosaccharide malabsorption. Acta Paediatr. 1962 Nov;51:674-85.

[8] Turk E, Zabel B, Mundlos S, Dyer J, Wright EM. Glucose/galactose malabsorption caused by a defect in the Na+/glucose cotransporter. Nature. 1991 Mar 28;350(6316): 354-6.

[9] van den Heuvel LP, Assink K, Willemsen M, Monnens L. Autosomal recessive renal glucosuria attributable to a mutation in the sodium glucose cotransporter (SGLT2). Hum Genet. 2002 Dec;111(6):544-7.

[10] Jurczak MJ, Lee HY, Birkenfeld AL, Jornayvaz FR, Frederick DW, Pongratz RL, et al. SGLT2 deletion improves glucose homeostasis and preserves pancreatic beta-cell function. Diabetes. 2011 2011;60(3):890-8.

[11] Rossetti L, Smith D, Shulman GI, Papachristou D, DeFronzo RA. Correction of hyperglycemia with phlorizin normalizes tissue sensitivity to insulin in diabetic rats. J Clin Invest. 1987 May;79(5):1510-5.

[12] Chao EC, Henry RR. SGLT2 inhibition--a novel strategy for diabetes treatment. Nat Rev Drug Discov. 2010 Jul;9(7):551-9.

[13] Bays H. Sodium Glucose Co-transporter Type 2 (SGLT2) Inhibitors: Targeting the Kidney to Improve Glycemic Control in Diabetes Mellitus. Diabetes Ther. 2013 Dec; 4(2):195-220.

[14] Diez-Sampedro A, Hirayama BA, Osswald C, Gorboulev V, Baumgarten K, Volk C, et al. A glucose sensor hiding in a family of transporters. Proc Natl Acad Sci U S A. 2003 Sep 30;100(20):11753-8.

[15] Faham S, Watanabe A, Besserer GM, Cascio D, Specht A, Hirayama BA, et al. The crystal structure of a sodium galactose transporter reveals mechanistic insights into Na+/sugar symport. Science. 2008 Aug 8;321(5890):810-4.

[16] Bianchi L, Diez-Sampedro A. A single amino acid change converts the sugar sensor SGLT3 into a sugar transporter. PLoS One. 2010;5(4):e10241.

[17] Kothinti RK, Blodgett AB, North PE, Roman RJ, Tabatabai NM. A novel SGLT is expressed in the human kidney. Eur J Pharmacol. 2012 Sep 5;690(1-3):77-83.

[18] Tazawa S, Yamato T, Fujikura H, Hiratochi M, Itoh F, Tomae M, et al. SLC5A9/SGLT4, a new Na+-dependent glucose transporter, is an essential transporter for mannose, 1,5-anhydro-D-glucitol, and fructose. Life Sci. 2005 Jan 14;76(9):1039-50.

[19] Grempler R, Augustin R, Froehner S, Hildebrandt T, Simon E, Mark M, et al. Functional characterisation of human SGLT-5 as a novel kidney-specific sodium-dependent sugar transporter. FEBS Lett. 2012 Feb 3;586(3):248-53.

[20] Fukuzawa T, Fukazawa M, Ueda O, Shimada H, Kito A, Kakefuda M, et al. SGLT5 reabsorbs fructose in the kidney but its deficiency paradoxically exacerbates hepatic steatosis induced by fructose. PLoS One. 2013;8(2):e56681.

[21] Bersudsky Y, Shaldubina A, Agam G, Berry GT, Belmaker RH. Homozygote inositol transporter knockout mice show a lithium-like phenotype. Bipolar Disord. 2008 Jun; 10(4):453-9.

[22] Coady MJ, Wallendorff B, Gagnon DG, Lapointe JY. Identification of a novel Na+/myo-inositol cotransporter. J Biol Chem. 2002 Sep 20;277(38):35219-24.

[23] Aouameur R, Da Cal S, Bissonnette P, Coady MJ, Lapointe JY. SMIT2 mediates all myo-inositol uptake in apical membranes of rat small intestine. Am J Physiol Gastrointest Liver Physiol. 2007 Dec;293(6):G1300-7.

[24] Lahjouji K, Aouameur R, Bissonnette P, Coady MJ, Bichet DG, Lapointe JY. Expression and functionality of the Na+/myo-inositol cotransporter SMIT2 in rabbit kidney. Biochim Biophys Acta. 2007 May;1768(5):1154-9.

[25] Wilson-O'Brien AL, Patron N, Rogers S. Evolutionary ancestry and novel functions of the mammalian glucose transporter (GLUT) family. BMC Evol Biol. 2010;10:152.

[26] Mueckler M, Caruso C, Baldwin SA, Panico M, Blench I, Morris HR, et al. Sequence and structure of a human glucose transporter. Science. 1985 Sep 6;229(4717):941-5.

[27] De Vivo DC, Trifiletti RR, Jacobson RI, Ronen GM, Behmand RA, Harik SI. Defective glucose transport across the blood-brain barrier as a cause of persistent hypoglycorrhachia, seizures, and developmental delay. N Engl J Med. 1991 Sep 5;325(10):703-9.

[28] Seidner G, Alvarez MG, Yeh JI, O'Driscoll KR, Klepper J, Stump TS, et al. GLUT-1 deficiency syndrome caused by haploinsufficiency of the blood-brain barrier hexose carrier. Nat Genet. 1998 Feb;18(2):188-91.

[29] Michau A, Guillemain G, Grosfeld A, Vuillaumier-Barrot S, Grand T, Keck M, et al. Mutations in SLC2A2 gene reveal hGLUT2 function in pancreatic beta cell development. J Biol Chem. 2013 Oct 25;288(43):31080-92.

[30] Sansbury FH, Flanagan SE, Houghton JA, Shuixian Shen FL, Al-Senani AM, Habeb AM, et al. SLC2A2 mutations can cause neonatal diabetes, suggesting GLUT2 may have a role in human insulin secretion. Diabetologia. 2012 Sep;55(9):2381-5.

[31] Seyer P, Vallois D, Poitry-Yamate C, Schutz F, Metref S, Tarussio D, et al. Hepatic glucose sensing is required to preserve beta cell glucose competence. J Clin Invest. 2013 Apr 1;123(4):1662-76.

[32] Tarussio D, Metref S, Seyer P, Mounien L, Vallois D, Magnan C, et al. Nervous glucose sensing regulates postnatal beta cell proliferation and glucose homeostasis. J Clin Invest. 2014 Jan 2;124(1):413-24.

[33] Coucke PJ, Willaert A, Wessels MW, Callewaert B, Zoppi N, De Backer J, et al. Mutations in the facilitative glucose transporter GLUT10 alter angiogenesis and cause arterial tortuosity syndrome. Nat Genet. 2006 Apr;38(4):452-7.

[34] Callewaert BL, Loeys BL, Casteleyn C, Willaert A, Dewint P, De Backer J, et al. Absence of arterial phenotype in mice with homozygous slc2A10 missense substitutions. Genesis. 2008 Aug;46(8):385-9.

[35] Cheng CH, Kikuchi T, Chen YH, Sabbagha NG, Lee YC, Pan HJ, et al. Mutations in the SLC2A10 gene cause arterial abnormalities in mice. Cardiovasc Res. 2009 Feb 1;81(2):381-8.

[36] Purcell SH, Aerni-Flessner LB, Willcockson AR, Diggs-Andrews KA, Fisher SJ, Moley KH. Improved insulin sensitivity by GLUT12 overexpression in mice. Diabetes. 2011 May;60(5):1478-82.

[37] Pujol-Gimenez J, Barrenetxe J, Gonzalez-Muniesa P, Lostao MP. The facilitative glucose transporter GLUT12: what do we know and what would we like to know? J Physiol Biochem. 2013 Jun;69(2):325-33.

[38] Manz F, Bickel H, Brodehl J, Feist D, Gellissen K, Gescholl-Bauer B, et al. Fanconi-Bickel syndrome. Pediatr Nephrol. 1987 Jul;1(3):509-18.

[39] Preitner F, Bonny O, Laverriere A, Rotman S, Firsov D, Da Costa A, et al. Glut9 is a major regulator of urate homeostasis and its genetic inactivation induces hyperuricosuria and urate nephropathy. Proc Natl Acad Sci U S A. 2009 Sep 8;106(36):15501-6.

Chapter 2

Structural and Functional Evolution of Glucose Transporter 4 (GLUT4): A Look at GLUT4 in Fish

Rubén Marín-Juez, Encarnación Capilla,
Francisco Carvalho-Simoes, Marta Camps and
Josep V. Planas

Additional information is available at the end of the chapter

http://dx.doi.org/10.5772/58094

1. Introduction

The insulin-responsive glucose transporter GLUT4 was first described in 1988 as a result of studies on the regulation of glucose metabolism by insulin [1]. Soon after the discovery of GLUT4, several groups cloned GLUT4 in the human [2], rat [3,4] and mouse [5]. Since its discovery, GLUT4 has received, together with GLUT1, more experimental attention than any other single membrane transport protein. Structurally, GLUT4 follows the predicted model for class I glucose transporters. GLUT4 has a high affinity for glucose, with a Km of approximately 5 mM [6], and also transports mannose, galactose, dehydroascorbic acid and glucosamine [7-10]. In mammals, GLUT4 is mainly expressed in cardiac and skeletal muscle, brown and white adipose tissue, and brain [6,11,12]. GLUT4 plays a pivotal role in whole body glucose homeostasis, mediating the uptake of glucose regulated by insulin [13,14]. GLUT4 is responsible for the reduction in the postprandial rise in plasma glucose levels [6]. Insulin acts by stimulating the translocation of specific GLUT4-containing vesicles from intracellular stores to the plasma membrane (PM) resulting in an immediate increase in glucose transport [6,15]. The disruption of GLUT4 expression has been extensively associated with pathologies of impaired glucose uptake and insulin resistance such as type 2 diabetes and obesity [13,16-18].

Glucose is a central molecule for the metabolism of all vertebrates and plays a pivotal role as fuel and metabolic substrate [19]. From an evolutionary perspective, the regulation of glucose metabolism in non-mammalian vertebrates appears to be slightly different than in mammals, particularly with respect to their tolerance of hyperglycemia (reviewed in [20]). A large body of research has been devoted to the study of glucose metabolism in fish species, mostly due to their phylogenetic position and their economic interest (i.e. fisheries and aquaculture). As a result of their lower ability to return to normoglycemia after feeding or after a glucose load, when compared to mammals, fish have been considered to be "glucose intolerant" [21]. This conclusion was based on the demonstrated lower ability of fish peripheral tissues (e.g. mostly the skeletal muscle, representing more than 50% of the body weight) to utilize glucose [22]. However, despite the low glucose uptake in the fish skeletal muscle, when compared to mammals, there was evidence indicating that skeletal muscle represents not only the main site of glucose uptake but that it was the only tissue in which the rate of glucose uptake was increased after a glucose load [23], suggesting that glucose uptake in skeletal muscle could be regulated. Given that insulin had been shown to lower blood glucose levels in fish by, at least in part, stimulating the *in vivo* uptake and utilization of glucose mostly by the skeletal muscle [24] and given that the blood levels of insulin were shown to be increased by administration of a glucose load in trout [23], it was hypothesized that insulin may exert its hypoglycemic effects in fish through the regulation of glucose transporters, possibly GLUT4. Initially it was claimed that GLUT4 did not exist in fish based on the inability of antibodies against mammalian GLUT4 to recognize a putative fish GLUT4 protein [25]. However, the identification of a true GLUT4 homolog in fish in 2000 by molecular cloning [26] paved the way for investigating the possible regulation of glucose homeostasis in fish through the regulation of an insulin-regulatable glucose transporter homologous to GLUT4. Here, we review the accumulated evidence to date on the functional characteristics and regulation of the GLUT4 homolog in fish.

2. Evolution of the structural characteristics of the GLUT4 gene

Among the sequenced genomes of vertebrate species, the GLUT4 gene (named SLC2A4) is found in mammals (41 species), reptiles (2 species) and ray-finned fishes (10 species) (Figure 1), suggesting that the GLUT4 gene has been conserved throughout evolution. Surprisingly, the GLUT4 gene is absent among birds and amphibians. The lack of GLUT4 in birds, but the presence of other GLUT family members (Glut1, Glut2 and Glut3), has recently been confirmed experimentally [27]. Moreover, no GLUT4 gene is present in the only amphibian genome available to date (i.e. *Xenopus tropicalis*) and searches for GLUT4 in Xenopus EST databases were unable to yield any transcript with homology for GLUT4. At this time, it is not known if the lack of the GLUT4 gene is general of the avian and amphibian classes, particularly since only a very reduced number of species have been examined, and, more importantly, if these two groups of vertebrates have subsequently lost the GLUT4 gene after their emergence.

http://dx.doi.org/10.5772/58094

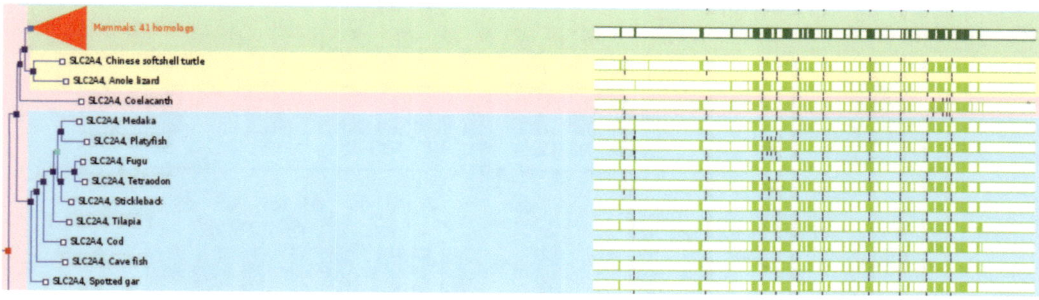

Figure 1. Evolutionary tree of the GLUT4 gene (SLC2A4) in vertebrates. Alignment of the different GLUT4 gene sequences is shown on the right. White sections of the alignment indicate gaps in the sequence.

2.1. Structural characteristics of the GLUT4 gene in fish

Fish, after mammals, are the vertebrate group for which more genomic information is available mainly due to their importance as research model species (e.g. medaka, zebrafish, stickleback) and for their economic importance in fisheries and aquaculture (e.g. cod, tilapia). Therefore, fish are only second to mammals in the number of species for which there is genomic information corresponding to the GLUT4 gene. In mammals, the GLUT4 gene is located in chromosome 17 and consists of 11 coding exons, spanning 6.6 kb. Despite the fact that the fish GLUT4 protein is well conserved among the different fish species (see section 3), certain structural differences among the fish GLUT4 genes can be observed. For example, the number of exons coding for GLUT4 and the length of the GLUT4 gene varies among the different species: 12 exons in Fugu, 13 in Tetraodon, 13 in Tilapia, 11 in Stickleback, 12 in Medaka and 15 in Platyfish, spanning 4.8 kb, 4.5 kb, 10.2 kb, 4.9 kb, 12.7 kb and 14.1 kb, respectively (Figure 2). Moreover, it is worth mentioning that exons 6 to 10 of the human GLUT4 gene appear to be highly conserved in fish (Figure 2). The only fish species with a sequenced genome for which the GLUT4 gene appears to be absent is the zebrafish. The lack of a GLUT4 gene in the zebrafish genome sequence database (Ensembl) is related to the lack of transcripts for GLUT4 in zebrafish EST dabases. These observations support the notion that zebrafish may have lost the GLUT4 gene.

In addition to the gene structure characteristics of GLUT4 in fish, another aspect of interest with regards to the evolution of GLUT4 is whether the genes flanking the GLUT4 loci in the genome of the various fish species have also been conserved. A synthetic analysis of the GLUT4 loci in different fish species evidences that a number of the genes flanking the fish GLUT4 genes are homologs to those flanking the human GLUT4 gene (e.g. YBX2, EIF5AL1, GPS2, GABARAP, CTDNEP1, NEURL4, TNK1, PLSCR3) (Figure 3A). Furthermore, the nature and the genomic position of the genes flanking the GLUT4 gene in fish are highly conserved across the different fish species (Figure 3B).

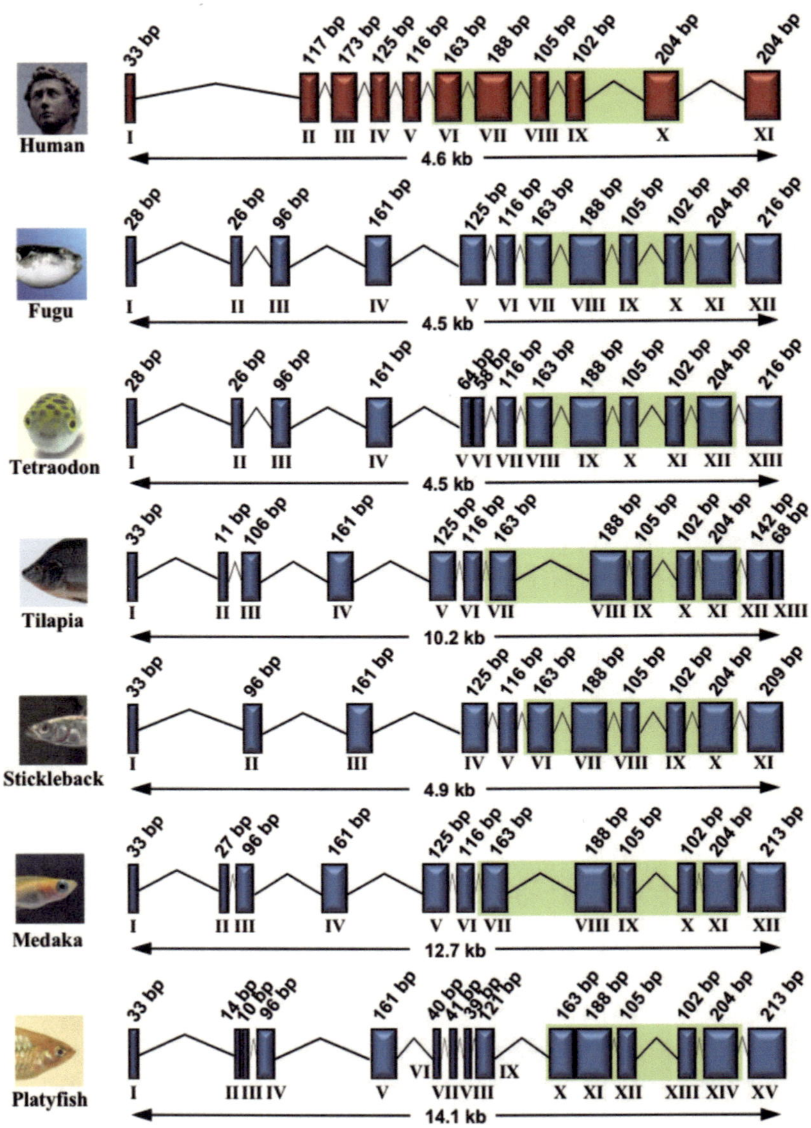

Figure 2. Genomic structure and organization of GLUT4 in fish. Exons are represented by solid boxes and introns are represented by connecting lines. The sizes of exons are shown in base pairs on the top of the boxes. Exons are numbered with roman numbers beneath the boxes. Exons conserved in all the species are highlighted in green. Gene IDs were retieved from public databases-Human: ENSG00000181856; Fugu: ENSTRUG00000011935; Tetraodon: ENSTNIG00000010138; Tilapia: ENSONIG00000018958; Stickleback: ENSGACG00000019384; Medaka: ENSORLG00000006341; Platyfish: ENSXMAG00000015723.

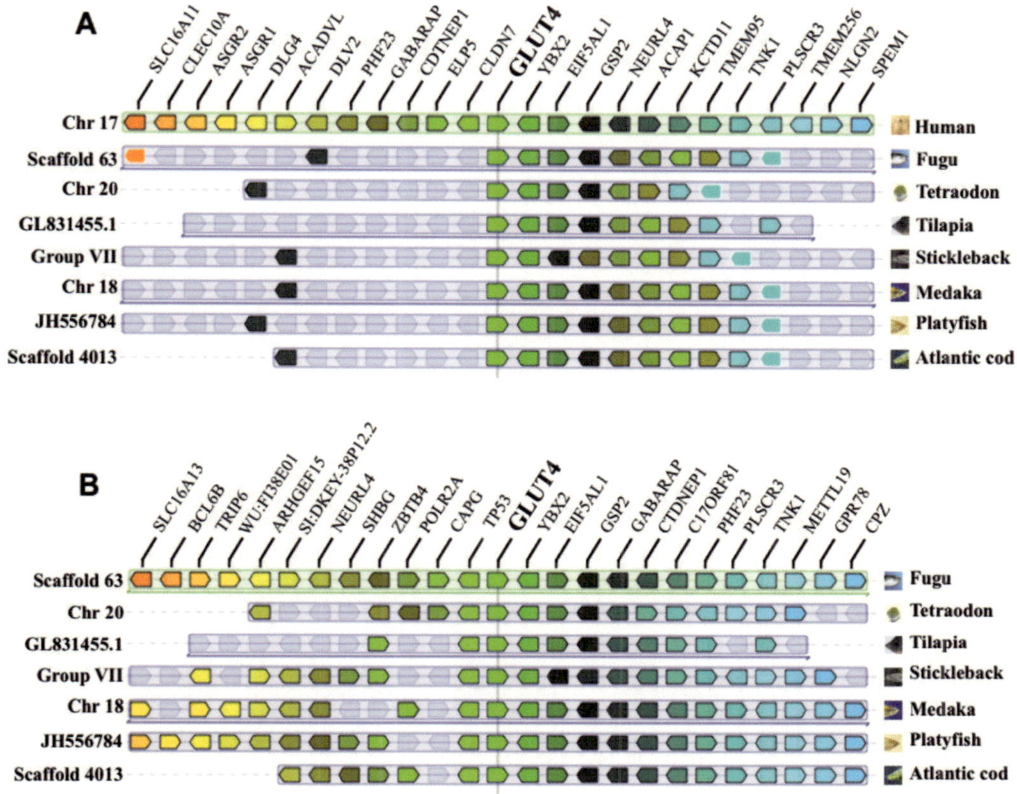

Figure 3. Comparison of genomic regions carrying GLUT4 loci. A. Synteny in relation to the human GLUT4 gene. B. Synteny of fish GLUT4 genes in relation to the Fugu GLUT4 gene. Boxes of the same color indicate the position of the ortholog in the different species. The coding direction of the genes is indicated by the pointed end. Pale blue symbols indicate nonsyntenic genes. Location in the Genome of each species is indicated at the left side of the diagram. Gene IDs were retrieved from public databases-Human: ENSG00000181856; Fugu: ENSTRUG00000011935; Tetraodon: ENSTNIG00000010138; Tilapia: ENSONIG00000018958; Stickleback: ENSGACG00000019384; Medaka: ENSORLG00000006341; Platyfish: ENSXMAG00000015723; Atlantic cod: ENSGMOG00000007757. The diagram was generated using Genomicus genome browser [28].

As is known in mammals, the GLUT4 gene undergoes an important regulation at the transcriptional level that takes place in the upstream regulatory regions of the gene (i.e. promoter region) [29]. Recently, the promoter region of the GLUT4 gene in a fish species (i.e. Fugu) was characterized for the first time [30]. A 1.3 kb 5′-flanking region of the Fugu GLUT4 gene was characterized with 3 possible transcription start sites, a conserved cluster of CpG dinucleoties (i.e. CpG island) and several transcription factor binding sites known to be important for the transcriptional regulation of the mammalian GLUT4 gene such as MEF2, SREBP, KLF, SP1/GC-box, NF-Y, E-box, PPARγ, PPAR-RXR and HIF-1 (Figure 4) [30]. In addition, like in mammals, the Fugu GLUT4 gene promoter lacks TATA-box elements [30]. *In silico* comparison of the 1.3 kb genomic DNA region upstream of the GLUT4 gene in different fish species revealed the presence of two highly conserved regions containing most of the above cited binding motifs (Figure 4). Interestingly, these two regions contain the E-box/MEF2/Klf cassette, which is an important cassette placed in an enhancer region of the promoter of the GLUT4 gene in mammals [29], and the core promoter, essential for the basal expression of the GLUT4 gene. These observations highlight the high degree of conservation of the GLUT4 gene and its regulatory region during evolution from fish to mammals.

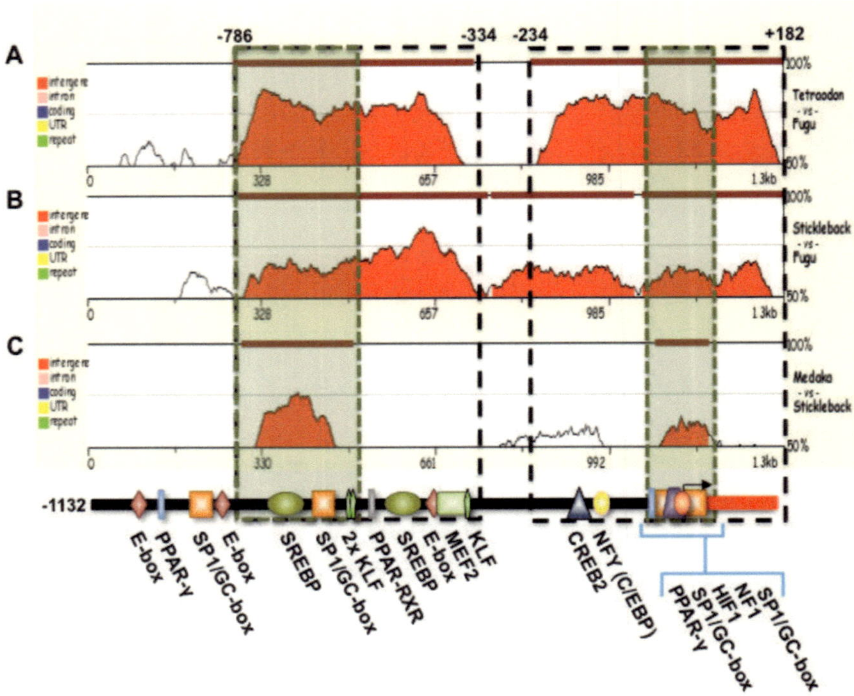

Figure 4. Conservation profile of the promoter region of known fish GLUT4 genes. Sequence elements of significant length (≥ 100 nucleotides) that show higher than 60% of homology are highlighted in red and depicted with the dark-red rectangles on the top of each graph. The sequence comparison between the Fugu and Tetraodon (A), Fugu and Stickleback (B) and Stickleback and Medaka (C) GLUT4 promoters is shown. The horizontal axis represents the position of the nucleotides within the 1314 bp sequence compared, starting at the 5′ end. The vertical axis represents the percent of identity between the aligned genomes. In the bottom, a schematic representation of the-1132 Fugu GLUT4 gene promoter highlighting the most relevant predicted binding sites is shown. The open boxes delineating the regions comprised between-786/-334 and-234/+182 nucleotides represent conserved areas in fish GLUT4 gene promoters. Adapted from [30].

3. Structural characteristics of the GLUT4 protein in fish

In fish, the deduced amino acid sequence of GLUT4 is known in approximately 10 different species as a result of either conventional cloning techniques or available sequences in databases. Similar to mammalian GLUT4, a protein of 509 amino acids in length, known fish GLUT4 proteins range between 503 and 511 amino acids in length. Also like mammalian GLUT4, fish GLUT4 proteins have a predicted molecular mass of approximately 55 kDa and an isoelectric point of 6.7. Western blotting using polyclonal antibodies against coho salmon GLUT4 (okGLUT4) confirmed that the molecular weight of native GLUT4 in adipose tissue and skeletal muscle cells from salmonid species was approximately 50 kDa [31,32]. Comparison of human GLUT4 and fish GLUT4 proteins evidences a relatively high degree of conservation at the amino acid level, with fish GLUT4 proteins showing a 79% sequence homology to human GLUT4. However, fish GLUT4 proteins show more than 90% homology amongst themselves at the amino acid level, even when considering species that are phylogenetically distant such as coho salmon and tilapia. Phylogenetic analyses of fish GLUT4 proteins in relation to human GLUT4 reveal that all fish GLUT4 proteins are evolutionarily related to human GLUT4 and that they cluster according to their phylogenetic position within the fish evolutionary tree (Figure 5).

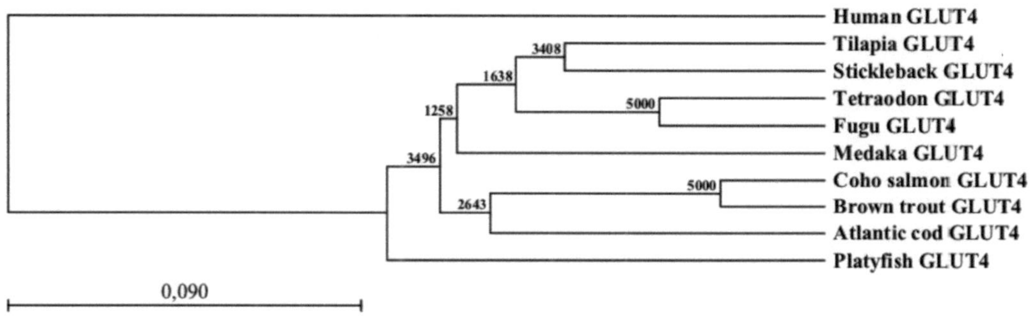

Figure 5. Unrooted phylogenetic tree of GLUT4 amino acid sequences. The tree was created by the UPGMA method using ClustalW multiple alignment and bootstrapped 5000 times. The scale for the given branch length indicates 0.09 amino acid substitutions per site. Gene IDs and accession numbers were retrieved from public databases-Human: ENSG00000181856; Fugu: ENSTRUG00000011935; Tetraodon: ENSTNIG00000010138; Tilapia: ENSONIG00000018958; Stickleback: ENSGACG00000019384; Medaka: ENSORLG00000006341; Platyfish: ENSXMAG00000015723; Atlantic cod: AAZ15731.1; Brown trout: AAG12191.1; Coho Salmon: AAM22227.1.

Importantly, the structural characteristics of all the known fish GLUT4 proteins correspond to those of the facilitated glucose transporter family and, specifically, to those of mammalian GLUT4. The structural conservation of GLUT4 from fish to mammals can clearly be observed when an alignment of the deduced amino acid sequence of fish GLUT4 proteins with human GLUT4 is performed (Figure 6). Like human GLUT4, all fish GLUT4 proteins contain the typical 12 (I-XII) hydrophobic transmembrane domains (TMs) of 21 amino acids that have also been revealed by hydropathy plots [26,31]. Furthermore, all fish GLUT4 proteins contain four major hydrophylic regions corresponding to the amino (N) terminus, the carboxy (C) terminus and the two main extracellular and intracellular domains. The main extracellular domain corresponds to a loop of approximately 30 amino acids located between TMI and TMII and contains a predicted glycosylation site (K^{50}) that is present in all mammalian and avian GLUT proteins. The large intracellular domain corresponds to a cytoplasmic loop of 65 amino acids located between TMVI and TMVII. Other structural characteristics of functional GLUT proteins that are found in fish GLUT4 include the presence of (1) the QLS motif in TMVII, known to be important for the high-affinity recognition of the transported substrate, (2) the

STS sequence in the extracellular segment between TMVII and TMVIII, known to be important for the conformational change of GLUT4 during the transport of glucose and (3) several proline (P) residues in TMVI and TMX that are known to be important for transport activity [33-35] (Figure 6).

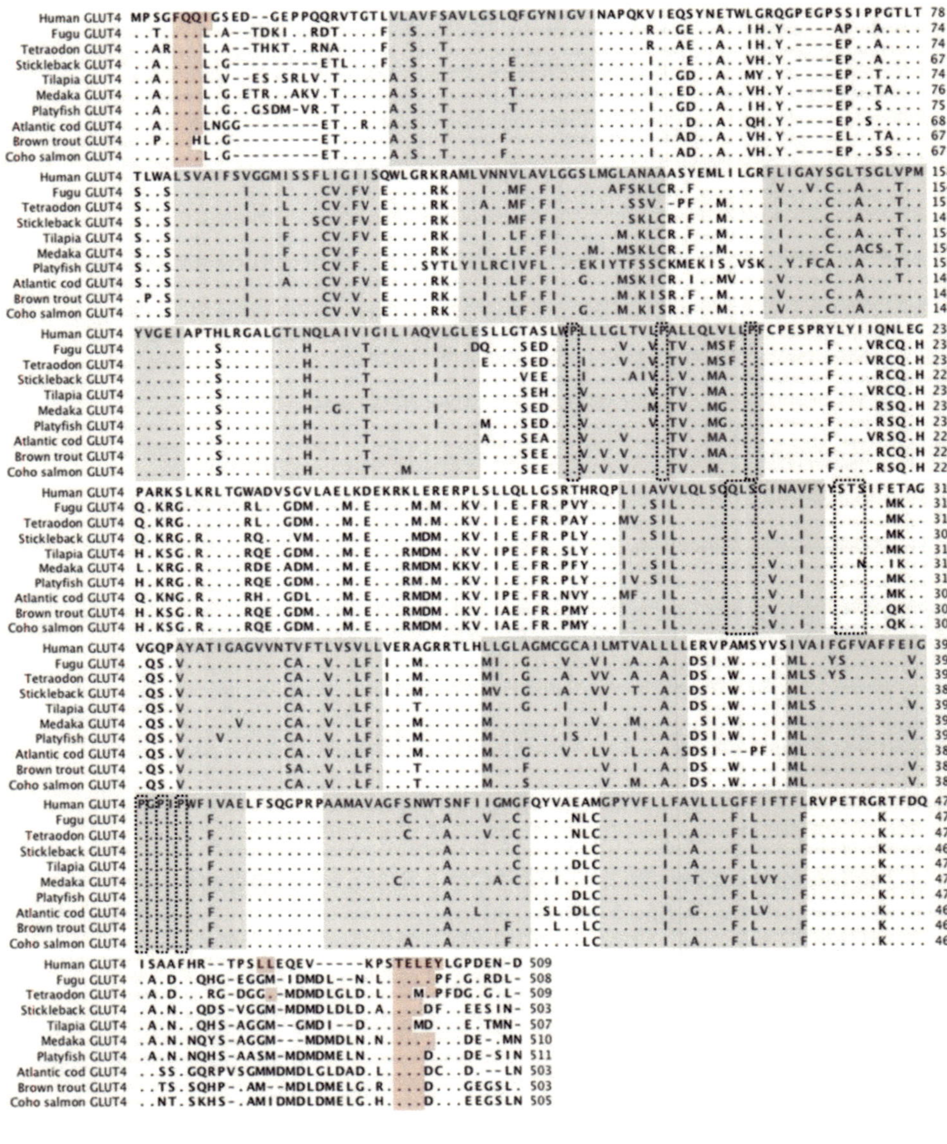

Figure 6. Multiple alignment of GLUT4 protein sequences. Identical residues identified using ClustalW are indicated as dots. Grey boxes: Transmembrane domains. Red boxes: Important motives for GLUT4 trafficking. Dashed box: Important motive for glucose transport. Gene IDs and accession numbers were retrieved from public databases-Human: ENSG00000181856; Fugu: ENSTRUG00000011935; Tetraodon: ENSTNIG00000010138; Tilapia: ENSONIG00000018958; Stickleback: ENSGACG00000019384; Medaka: ENSORLG00000006341; Platyfish: ENSXMAG00000015723; Atlantic cod: AAZ15731.1; Brown trout: AAG12191.1; Coho Salmon: AAM22227.1.

In addition to having sequence features typical of GLUTs, fish GLUT4 proteins also share certain sequence motifs that are characteristic of GLUT4 and that confer its particular intracellular traffic behavior. Specifically, the N-terminus of human GLUT4 contains the F^5QQI^8 motif that has been shown to be important for its internalization from the cell surface [36]. Furthermore, the C-terminus of human GLUT4 contains the acidic cluster $T^{498}ELEY^{502}$ that has been shown to be important for the intracellular retention of GLUT4 under basal conditions [37] (see below). Mutations of either these two motifs in GLUT4 lead to alterations in the intracellular traffic of GLUT4 [37]. Importantly, fish GLUT4 proteins contain these two essential motifs, although with some differences in their sequence. For example, fish GLUT4 proteins show similarities to human GLUT4 in terms of the sequence of these two motifs. The F^5QQI^8 motif is present in the form of F^5QQL^8 in all fish species examined, except for brown trout (btGLUT4) that has a F^5QHL^8 motif (Figure 6). As will be discussed below, substitution of H^7 for Q^7 may have functional consequences for the traffic of GLUT4 among the different fish species. In addition, the $T^{498}ELEY^{502}$ motif is present in fish GLUT4 proteins, with medaka GLUT4 having an identical motif but with small substitutions in other fish GLUT4 proteins, such as D^{501} for E^{501} in six species (i.e. salmon, trout, cod, platyfish, tilapia and stickleback) and such as M^{500} for L^{500} in only two species (tetraodon and tilapia). The C-terminal residue Y^{502}, thought to be important for regulating the release of GLUT4 from its intracellular storage compartments [38], was present in five of the fish species examined (tilapia, medaka, platyfish, trout and salmon). However, despite these similarities between human and fish GLUT4 proteins, the motif $L^{489}L^{490}$ that is thought to be important for the regulation of GLUT4 translocation from cytosolic compartments to the PM and for its endocytosis [39-41], is not present in fish GLUT4 proteins. Therefore, although fish GLUT4 proteins are clearly homologous to mammalian GLUT4 and contain protein motifs important for the function, regulation and traffic of GLUT4, they show differences in the sequence of these important motifs that may account for slightly different properties. One interesting possibility is that the above-mentioned differences in the primary structure between fish and mammalian GLUT4 could cause differences in the structure/conformation of the transporter, which could affect its ability to transport glucose and/or to bind factors that interact with GLUT4 and, consequently, alter its intracellular traffic. For this reason, studies have been performed with fish GLUT4 as a natural mutant of mammalian GLUT4 to contribute to our understanding of the role of the specific domains of GLUT4 that are responsible for its traffic behavior (see Section 6).

4. Sugar transport properties of fish GLUT4

The functionality of GLUT4 in fish has been investigated for okGLUT4 using the *Xenopus laevis* oocyte system [31]. The *Xenopus* oocyte system was extensively used in the 90s to functionally characterize the different GLUT isoforms in mammals [7,8,42,43], since it presents a series of advantages with respect to other *in vitro* systems: 1) the oocyte contains all the machinery necessary to properly express heterologous proteins; 2) it has very low endogenous levels of glucose transport, which avoids interferences in the measurements; and 3) it allows to analyze separately GLUTs that *in vivo* may be present together in the same tissue. Therefore, using this system, okGLUT4 was demonstrated to be a functional glucose transporter, with characteristics similar to those of its mammalian counterparts [31].

Regarding the kinetics of fish GLUT4, studies were performed using zero-trans and equilibrium exchange conditions with 2-deoxy-glucose (2-DG) and the non-metabolizable glucose analogue, 3-O-methylglucose (3-OMG), respectively [31]. From the zero-trans kinetic analyses, the transport of glucose by the oocyte was demonstrated to be saturable, with a Km value on average of 7.6 mM. Using the equilibrium exchange assay and, assuming the transport follows first-order kinetics, the average Km value calculated for 3-OMG uptake by okGLUT4-expressing oocytes was of 14.4 mM. These Km values were higher than those reported using the same oocyte system for mammalian GLUT4s: 4.6 and 1.8-4.3 mM for zero-trans and equilibrium exchange kinetics, respectively [7,8,44], suggesting that the fish transporter has less affinity for glucose. Nevertheless, when compared with kinetics of the Glut1 isoform identified in trout (OnmyGlut1), also studied in *Xenopus* oocytes, we observed that the zero-trans Km value of okGLUT4 was lower than that of OnmyGlut1 (8.3-14.9 mM) [45]. Moreover, the Km value reported in American eel erythrocytes, that primarily express Glut1, was also higher (10.4 mM) than that of okGLUT4 [46]; thus, indicating that the relative affinity for glucose of fish GLUTs parallels that of mammals, since the ubiquitous Glut1 has also lower affinity for glucose (21.3-26.2 mM) than GLUT4 [7,44]. On the other hand, the lower affinity for glucose of the fish GLUTs in comparison to mammals, may explain the reduced tolerance presented by the former to dietary carbohydrates [21,22].

To further characterize the fish GLUT4 transporter, stereoselectivity and substrate specificity were also analyzed in *Xenopus* oocytes expressing okGLUT4, using different sugars as transport competitors of 2-DG [31]. okGLUT4 was demonstrated to be stereospecific as its mammalian counterparts [8,31], since all the D-monosaccharides tested (glucose, mannose and galactose), but not the corresponding L-isomers, reduced the uptake of 2-DG into the oocyte. Interestingly, okGLUT4 transported all the various D-sugars, although with different affinities, as shown by the degree of competition towards 2-DG uptake observed for each monosaccharide. In this sense, D-glucose and D-mannose were primarily transported by okGLUT4 and, to a lesser extent, D-galactose and also D-fructose, albeit with even lower affinity. Overall, these data indicate that fish GLUT4 shows lower substrate specificity than mammalian GLUT4, suggesting that they may have a broader range of functions in fish controlling glucose metabolism. In this sense, it is interesting to note that okGLUT4 is able to uptake fructose, a role that is attributed to Glut2 in mammals [8,31]. Therefore, together with the fact that fish GLUT4 has a wider tissue distribution, the transport characteristics of fish GLUT4 support the idea that GLUT4 may play a role in the postprandial absorption of dietary glucose.

Moreover, okGLUT4 transport activity was shown to be suppressed by different transport inhibitors; thus, corroborating that this fish transporter belongs to the family of facilitative GLUTs [31]. 2-DG uptake in *Xenopus* oocytes expressing okGLUT4 was dose-dependently decreased by the well-known intracellular inhibitor cytochalasin B [47-49] as well as by the extracellular inhibitor, ethylidene glucose [34]. Cytochalasin B was previously shown to inhibit glucose transport in fish erythrocytes, suggesting the existence of GLUT transporters in fish before their discovery [46,50-52], and later also in *Xenopus* oocytes expressing the OnmyGlut1 transporter [45]. Furthermore, in L6 muscle cells stably expressing btGLUT4, a dose-dependent inhibition in response to cytochalasin B was also reported [32]. In this same study, the effect of indinavir, a known GLUT4 mammalian inhibitor [53-55] was analyzed, causing also a concentration-dependent decrease on 2-DG uptake. Overall, these results confirm that okGLUT4 presents similar biochemical properties as mammalian GLUT4. In summary, all these studies have demonstrated that fish GLUT4 is a functional GLUT that is a structural and functional homolog of mammalian GLUT4 but with the important difference that has lower affinity for glucose and wider substrate specificity than mammalian GLUT4.

5. Regulation of the expression of GLUT4 in fish

As all membrane solute carriers, GLUT4 exerts its glucose transport properties when is present in the PM, allowing the flux of glucose across a concentration gradient. Therefore, the GLUT4-mediated transport of glucose can be determined, at least in great part, by the number of transporter molecules present at the PM at any given time. In mammals, the abundance of GLUT4 at the PM of skeletal muscle or adipose cells is, in turn, dependent on the traffic mechanisms that translocate pre-existing, vesicle-bound GLUT4 to the PM but, ultimately, on the synthesis of GLUT4 proteins (reviewed in [29]). The following section reviews available data on the regulation of fish GLUT4 at the mRNA, protein and promoter activity levels.

5.1. Regulation of GLUT4 mRNA levels in fish

In mammals, GLUT4 is mainly expressed in insulin-sensitive tissues, namely skeletal and cardiac muscle and adipose tissue. In skeletal muscle, GLUT4 is the main transporter expressed and it has been estimated that it accounts for approximately 70% of the basal glucose transport in this tissue (reviewed in [29]). In fish, the pattern of the tissue expression of GLUT4 at the mRNA level has only been examined in two different species: the brown trout [26] and the Atlantic cod [56]. In these two fish species, the level of GLUT4 mRNA was shown to be highest in red (slow) and white (fast) skeletal muscle. In Atlantic cod, the heart also showed high levels of GLUT4 mRNA but not in brown trout. Lower levels of GLUT4 mRNA were observed in adipose tissue, gill, kidney and other tissues in these two species. In rainbow trout, GLUT4 mRNA transcripts have also been detected in white skeletal muscle [57]. Overall, the pattern of tissue expression of GLUT4 transcripts in fish agrees well with the reported main expression of GLUT4 in the mammalian skeletal muscle, coinciding with this tissue as the primary insulin target and major site for glucose disposal. The presence of the GLUT4 protein in skeletal muscle and adipose tissue of trout has been confirmed by immunoblotting [31,32].

The expression of the GLUT4 gene is known to be subjected to an important transcriptional regulation that determines the protein levels of GLUT4 in skeletal and cardiac muscle and in adipose tissue in mammals. In mammals, a number of factors are known to influence GLUT4 expression, most notably the nutritional and dietary status and hormones (e.g. insulin, insulin-like growth factor I (IGF-I) and thyroid hormones) (reviewed in [28,58]). In fish, most current evidence regarding the regulation of GLUT4 expression is at the mRNA level and in skeletal muscle, due to the importance of this tissue in glucose homeostasis. As in mammals, the expression of GLUT4 mRNA levels increase during muscle cell differentiation in trout, as was demonstrated by the gradual increase in GLUT4 mRNA levels during the differentiation process of trout muscle cells in culture from myoblasts to myotubes [59]. In addition, the amount of immunoreactive GLUT4 was observed to be higher in trout myotubes than in myoblasts [32], strongly suggesting that GLUT4 can be considered a marker of muscle differentiation also in fish.

5.1.1. Regulation of GLUT4 mRNA levels by insulin in fish

In mammals, insulin exerts its hypoglycemic action in part by increasing the expression of GLUT4 in skeletal muscle. Data in fish also indicates that the expression of GLUT4 mRNA in skeletal muscle appears to be regulated by circulating insulin levels in a muscle type specific manner. As it is well known, fish skeletal muscle can be differentiated into two anatomically and functionally different types of muscle: white muscle, that is a fast, anaerobic muscle that permits sudden bursts of motion, and red muscle, that is a slow, aerobic muscle that permits sustained locomotion. Although red muscle only comprises 5-10% of the body weight in fish (in contrast to > 50% for white muscle), it has a higher glucose uptake rate and insulin receptor density than white muscle. Interestingly, the *in vivo* regulation of GLUT4 mRNA levels by circulating insulin in trout appears to take place only in red skeletal muscle. Decreases in circulating insulin levels caused by fasting or by feeding a diet containing low protein and high carbohydrate levels were associated with a decrease in GLUT4 mRNA levels in red but not white skeletal muscle in trout [60]. In contrast, increases in circulating insulin levels caused by insulin or arginine (an insulin secretagogue in fish; [24]) administration were accompanied by an increase in GLUT4 mRNA levels in red but not white skeletal muscle in trout [60]. More recently, it was shown that GLUT4 expression in white skeletal muscle of trout fed a diet rich in carbohydrates was not affected [57]. Therefore, there is strong evidence suggesting that GLUT4 mRNA levels in red skeletal muscle may be regulated *in vivo* by circulating insulin in trout, as in mammals. However, these observations raised the question as to whether the expression of GLUT4 could be regulated in white skeletal muscle, given that it accounts for the bulk of glucose taken up by skeletal muscle. In contrast to trout, GLUT4 mRNA levels in the white muscle of Atlantic cod increased after fasting and decreased after refeeding [56], suggesting the possibility of species-specific differences in the regulation of GLUT4 in this tissue.

In vitro studies using a primary culture of trout skeletal muscle cells have assessed the effects of insulin and IGF-I on GLUT4 mRNA levels. The results obtained from these studies clearly showed that insulin and IGF-I increased the GLUT4 mRNA content in myoblasts and in myotubes [59] and support the notion that insulin can indeed regulate GLUT4 mRNA levels in trout skeletal muscle by acting directly on muscle cells. Since insulin is known to stimulate the uptake of glucose by trout skeletal muscle cells *in vitro* [32], it has been hypothesized that this effect of insulin may have been due, at least in part, to its effects on GLUT4 expression. Therefore, it appears that the hypoglycemic effects of insulin in fish, as in mammals, may involve the stimulation of GLUT4 mRNA expression in skeletal muscle.

5.1.2. Regulation of GLUT4 mRNA levels by contractile activity in fish

In mammals, exercise is known to increase the transcription of the GLUT4 gene and, consequently, to increase glucose utilization in skeletal muscle [61,62]. The exercise-induced GLUT4 mRNA expression in the mammalian skeletal muscle is believed to be mediated largely by AMP-dependent protein kinase (AMPK), an energy sensor that is activated when increases in the AMP/ATP ratio occur, as in response to exercise [63]. In trout, swimming-induced exercise was also recently shown to promote glucose uptake and utilization in skeletal muscle [64]. Importantly, swimming-induced exercise increased the mRNA levels of GLUT4 in red and white skeletal muscle in trout, as in mammals [65], supporting the notion that the increase in GLUT4 in skeletal muscle may have been responsible, at least in part, for the decrease in circulating glucose levels and increased uptake and utilization of glucose by skeletal muscle of exercised trout [64]. Furthermore, pharmacological activation of AMPK by AICAR or metformin in trout skeletal muscle cells in culture caused an increase in GLUT4 mRNA levels [66]. Given that swimming-induced exercise increased AMPK activity in red and white skeletal muscle in trout (Magnoni and Planas, unpublished observations), there is strong evidence to believe that swimming-induced exercise increases GLUT4 mRNA levels in skeletal muscle through the induction of AMPK activity.

5.2. Regulation of the activity of the fish GLUT4 promoter

It is known that changes in the mRNA levels of GLUT4 in skeletal muscle in mammals (i.e. increases during exercise and decreases during states of insulin deficiency) are due to alterations in the transcription rate of the GLUT4 gene [29]. In mammals, the cis-regulatory region of the GLUT4 gene is relatively well characterized and is known to contain motifs that are important for the tissue-specific expression of the GLUT4 gene and its regulation. As indicated above (section 5.1.1), one of the most effective inducers of GLUT4 mRNA and protein expression in mammals is insulin. However, the regulation of the transcription of the GLUT4 gene by insulin in mammals is not well understood, particularly in the light of published data indicating that, paradoxically, insulin inhibits the transcription of the GLUT4 gene [67,68]. Interestingly, a recent study reported that the activity of a fish (i.e. Fugu) GLUT4 promoter, when expressed in mammalian muscle L6 cells, is inhibited by insulin [30]. Although the mechanism by which insulin represses the activity of the GLUT4 gene is not known in mammals, deletion analyses of the Fugu GLUT4 promoter have indicated that the region of the Fugu GLUT4 gene that is downstream of the main transcription start site may be sufficient for mediating the inhibitory effects of insulin on GLUT4 transcription [30]. Further studies are clearly needed to resolve the question of the paradoxical effects of insulin on GLUT4 gene transcription. Despite the inhibition of the activity of the Fugu GLUT4 gene promoter by insulin, other stimuli known to increase GLUT4 mRNA levels have been shown to cause an induction of Fugu GLUT4 promoter activity. First, ligand activation of PPARγ, which in mammals results in an increase of GLUT4 mRNA levels [69], increased the activity of the Fugu GLUT4 promoter expressed in L6 cells [30]. Second, electrical stimulation of mouse C2C12 myotubes expressing the Fugu GLUT4 promoter resulted in an increase in the activity of the Fugu GLUT4 promoter. Given the recent demonstration that swimming-induced skeletal muscle activity in trout increased the mRNA levels of GLUT4 in trout skeletal muscle [65], these results suggest that induction of contractile activity in skeletal muscle cells results in the transcriptional activation of the GLUT4 gene, resulting in increased GLUT4 mRNA levels that, in turn, may increase the amount of GLUT4 and, consequently, the entry and utilization of glucose in skeletal muscle in fish.

5.3. Regulation of GLUT4 protein levels in fish

To date, studies on the regulation of GLUT4 protein levels in fish are limited to salmonid species. The availability of a polyclonal antibody against okGLUT4 made possible the localization and the quantification of GLUT4 in trout skeletal muscle. By performing immunolocalization studies of GLUT4 in trout skeletal muscle cells in culture, an increase in the amount of total GLUT4 protein was observed during the differentiation of myoblasts into myotubes [32]. Subsequent studies showed that the total content of GLUT4 differs between the two types of skeletal muscle in trout, with red muscle containing a higher amount of GLUT4 than white muscle [70]. In agreement with changes in the expression of GLUT4 at the mRNA level, the total amount of GLUT4 protein in red muscle increased in trout stimulated with insulin *in vivo* and decreased after fasting. On the other hand, insulin administration failed to increase GLUT4 protein content in trout white muscle [32], supporting the lack of changes of GLUT4 mRNA levels previously described [60]. Interestingly, nutritional factors regulate GLUT4 mRNA and protein levels in white muscle in different manners. In trout, fasting decreased the amount of GLUT4 protein in white muscle [32], whereas no changes in mRNA levels were observed in the same condition [60], suggesting that post-transcriptional regulation of GLUT4 expression may take place in white skeletal muscle in fish. Therefore, it appears that insulin plasma levels may regulate the amount of GLUT4 present in red skeletal muscle in fish and strongly suggest that insulin may stimulate the de novo synthesis of GLUT4, at least in red skeletal muscle, by increasing the mRNA levels of GLUT4. The lack of effects after insulin administration *in vivo* on GLUT4 mRNA and protein levels in white muscle in trout are puzzling in the light of data showing that glucose uptake increases in white muscle after a glucose load in trout and that this tissue contributes about five times more than red muscle to the total glucose uptake when expressed as percent of the total body mass [23]. Further studies are required to understand the factors and mechanisms involved in the regulation of glucose uptake in white skeletal muscle in fish.

As part of the complex regulation of GLUT4, the translocation of this glucose transporter to the PM from intracellular vesicles is highly dynamic and is regulated by a number of factors [71], representing an efficient mechanism that allows a fast equilibration of glucose levels at either side of the PM in response to a hypoglycemic stimulus. In fish, insulin has been shown to increase the PM levels of GLUT4 in *in vitro* stimulated trout muscle cells in culture [32], demonstrating that insulin stimulates glucose uptake in fish skeletal muscle cells by increasing the levels of the GLUT4 protein at the PM, as in mammals. Other stimuli that have been shown to increase the uptake of glucose by trout myocytes and that also increase the cell surface levels of GLUT4 are AMPK activators (i.e. AICAR and metformin) [66] and the pro-inflammatory cytokine tumor necrosis factor α (TNFα) [72]. These results indicate that the regulation of the total amount of GLUT4 protein in skeletal muscle and, more importantly, the cell surface levels of GLUT4 in skeletal muscle cells are similar between fish and mammals, evidencing a remarkable degree of conservation of the mechanism(s) by which insulin exerts its hypoglycemic effects on skeletal muscle.

6. Regulation of the traffic of fish GLUT4

In mammals, the main feature that characterizes GLUT4 in skeletal muscle and adipose tissue and makes it unique is its ability to translocate to the PM in response to insulin [15,73]. This greatly increases the capacity of the cells to uptake glucose during the postprandial state, which is crucial to properly maintain glucose homeostasis. Notwithstanding, evidence in mammalian cells clearly indicates that in the basal state GLUT4 is not static; instead, GLUT4 circulates among numerous intracellular compartments, such as the trans-Golgi network (TGN), early and late endosomes, a specialized insulin responsive compartment (IRC), as well as the PM [71,74-75]. The amount of GLUT4 present at the PM in the basal state corresponds to about only 5-10% of the total GLUT4 protein, whereas the remaining 90-95% is sequestered intracellularly in the IRC compartment [76-78].

The intracellular trafficking characteristics of the two glucose transporters identified in salmonids (btGLUT4 and okGLUT4) have been studied in comparison with mammalian GLUT4 mainly when expressed in heterologous systems (mammalian adipocytic or myoblastic cell lines), but also as the endogenous GLUT4 in primary cultured trout myocytes. In 3T3-L1 adipocytes transiently expressing separately btGLUT4 or okGLUT4 under steady-state conditions, btGLUT4 exhibited significantly higher protein levels at the PM (30-40%), also okGLUT4 but to a lesser extent (15-20%), than rat GLUT4 (10-15%) [31,79]. This was not only observed in adipocytes, since btGLUT4 was present also at the PM at higher levels (20-25%) than rat GLUT4 (10-15%) when stably-expressed in L6 muscle cells [32]. Importantly, the basal localization of endogenous GLUT4 at the PM in trout myocytes in culture was also relatively high [32]. Therefore, under basal or unstimulated conditions fish GLUT4 appears to be less efficiently retained in the cytosol in adipocytes and myocytes than mammalian GLUT4, suggesting differences in the mechanisms responsible for the intracellular retention of GLUT4 between fish and mammals (see below). Furthermore, based on the observed differences in PM localization between fish GLUT4s under basal conditions, with okGLUT4 being more similar to its mammalian counterparts than btGLUT4, it has been suggested that the different traffic behavior of these two fish GLUT4 protein variants may be related to differences in characteristic regulatory features in the GLUT4 protein sequence (i.e. N-and C-terminal protein motifs) (see section 3; [79]).

Moreover, the ability of fish GLUT4s to respond to insulin has been also evaluated. The first studies trying to demonstrate that a fish GLUT4 translocates to the PM upon insulin stimulation were performed in *Xenopus* oocytes [31]. Nevertheless, the system was not appropriate to study the translocation of GLUT4 and oocytes expressing okGLUT4 or a rat GLUT4 did not show differences in transporter localization within the cell in response to insulin [31]. Instead, the 3T3-L1 adipocyte cell system was used successfully to demonstrate that both okGLUT4 and btGLUT4 were able to significantly translocate to the PM after insulin treatment [31,79], as it occurs in mammals. Moreover, insulin-stimulated translocation to the PM of btGLUT4 was demonstrated in L6 myoblasts and differentiated myotubes stably-expressing the fish GLUT4 transporter [32]. Therefore, the fish homologs of GLUT4 were shown to be insulin responsive like their mammalian counterpart, despite their higher PM localization at steady-state.

As previously mentioned, GLUT4 in mammals is distributed inside the cells in two major storage compartments, the IRC and the endosomal system [75,80]. Interestingly, btGLUT4 showed only partial co-localization with rat GLUT4 when both were co-expressed either in 3T3-L1 adipocytes [79] or in L6 muscle cells [32]. This observation, together with the fact that btGLUT4 showed lower levels of retention in intracellular compartments during basal conditions although it still responded to insulin stimulation in both cell types [32,79], suggested that btGLUT4 is equally distributed between the specialized IRC and the endosomal compartment, from where it cycles continuously with the PM. Moreover, both in 3T3-L1 adipocytes and L6 muscle cells, the higher PM levels observed for btGLUT4 were shown to be due to a faster externalization rate rather than to a decrease in the rate of endocytosis [32,79].

In mammals, several proteins have been described to interact with GLUT4 to regulate its intracellular traffic and to maintain the proteins sequestered in the IRC. For example, the Golgi-localized γ-ear-containing Arf-binding protein (GGA) has been described to function as a traffic controller of newly synthesized GLUT4 from the TGN to the IRC [73,81]. In this step, sortilin has been described also to have a key role, as GLUT4 does not contain the specific targeting motif to be recognized by GGA as a cargo molecule [82]. More recently, the insulin-regulated aminopeptidase (IRAP), which co-localizes with GLUT4 in intracellular vesicles, has been shown to play a role in the sorting of GLUT4 from endosomes into the IRC [83]. Moreover, a protein named TUG (tether containing a UBX domain for GLUT4), has been reported to interact with the large intracellular GLUT4 loop present between TMVI and TMVII and to tether GLUT4 to intracellular vesicles through its interaction, via its UBX domain, with cellular membranes [84]. The possible roles of several GLUT4-interacting proteins in the regulation of the traffic of the fish GLUT4 isoforms have been explored in 3T3-L1 adipocytes expressing the corresponding mammalian orthologs. In particular, the adaptor protein GGA has been reported to be involved in the early sorting steps of GLUT4 from the TGN. The expression in 3T3-L1 adipocytes of rat GLUT4 together with wild-type GGA or a dominant-interfering form of GGA (GGA-DN) demonstrated that GGA is required for GLUT4 to reach the IRC because the insulin-stimulated translocation of rat GLUT4 to the PM was completely blunted in the presence of GGA-DN [40,73]. Interestingly, the intracellular traffic of btGLUT4 and okGLUT4 in 3T3-L1 adipocytes showed differences with regards their sensitivities to GGA because the traffic of btGLUT4 to the PM either under basal or insulin-stimulated conditions was only partially suppressed by co-expression with GGA-DN whereas okGLUT4 showed an identical response as that of rat GLUT4 [79]. These results suggested that okGLUT4 may traffic in adipocytes through the same pathway as mammalian GLUT4, but that btGLUT4 may be in part escaping the regulated biosynthetic traffic route, moving to the PM following a GGA-independent pathway. In agreement with the different intracellular distribution observed between btGLUT4 and rat GLUT4 [32], the traffic of btGLUT4 to the PM may be occurring via the constitutive pathway used by Glut1 or the transferrin receptor [37,73] (Figure 7). It is known that GLUT4, upon arriving in the IRC, acquires the capability to respond to insulin and to translocate to the PM. When a plasmid coding rat GLUT4 is transfected into 3T3-L1 adipocytes, the cells require 6 to 9 hours to produce the new protein and to target it to the IRC [73,85]. In contrast, both okGLUT4 and btGLUT4, when expressed in the same cellular system, undergo insulin-stimulated translocation only 3 hours after transfection [79], suggesting that fish GLUT4 undergoes faster synthesis, processing or traffic. Interestingly, okGLUT4 showed a temporal response that was intermediate between rat GLUT4 and btGLUT4, but closer to the latter, despite showing a similar sensitivity towards GGA as the mammalian GLUT4.

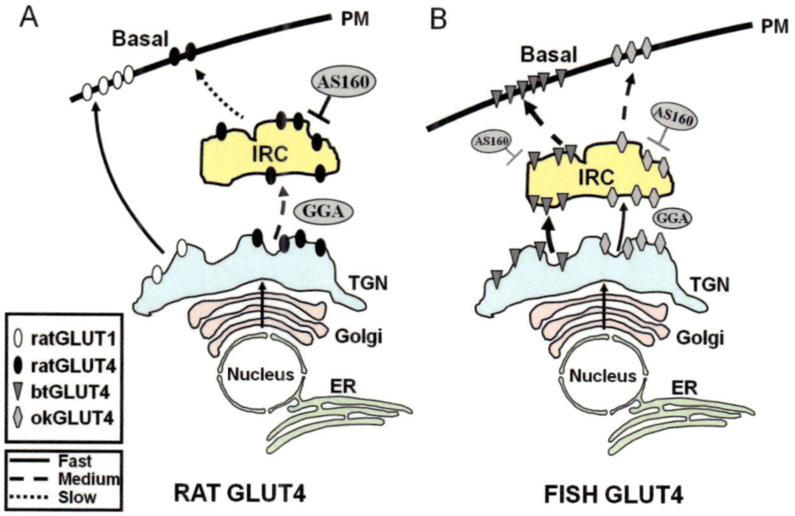

Figure 7. Schematic model illustrating differences in traffic between fish GLUT4s and rat GLUT4 and Glut1 during the basal state in adipocytes. In (A), the traffic of newly synthesized rat GLUT4 is shown to take place through the Golgi and the trans-Golgi network (TGN) and into the insulin-responsive compartment (IRC) in a sorting process that is dependent upon the adaptor protein GGA. In the basal state, rat GLUT4 is mainly sequestered into the IRC, a process that is regulated by AS160 and that requires the F^5QQI^8 amino terminal motif of GLUT4. In contrast, after biosynthesis, Glut1 directly travels from the TGN to the plasma membrane (PM) in a GGA-independent process. In (B), the traffic of newly synthesized trout (btGLUT4) or salmon (okGLUT4) GLUT4 is shown. We postulate that the high levels of btGLUT4 at the PM appear to be due to an increased exocytic rate, as a result of btGLUT4 following a GGA-independent route from the TGN to the IRC and by showing less AS160-regulated sequestration at the IRC than rat GLUT4. We hypothesize that the different trafficking behavior of btGLUT4 may be related to the different sequence in its N-terminal motif (F^5QHL^8). The traffic behavior of okGLUT4 (F^5QQL^8) appears to be intermediate between that of rat GLUT4 and btGLUT4. ER: endoplasmic reticulum.

As previously mentioned in section 3, among the different regulatory amino acid motifs found in GLUT4 in mammals, the F^5QQI^8 targeting motif in the N-terminus has been shown to be important for GLUT4 sequestration into the IRC and insulin-stimulated translocation to the PM [85-88]. Interestingly, in addition to the fact that both fish GLUT4 transporters have a shorter N-terminal domain, the F^5QQI^8 motif shows one conserved amino acid substitution in okGLUT4 (F^5QQL^8), and it is less conserved in btGLUT4 (F^5QHL^8), where the double residue substitution causes important size and charge changes (Figure 8A). The possibility that these sequence differences were able to account for the increased basal cell surface levels observed for btGLUT4 was investigated (Capilla and Planas, unpublished data). Figure 8B shows that mutation of the btGLUT4 motif F^5QHL^8 to F^5QQI^8 caused a slight decrease in basal PM levels; however, mutation of the F^5QHL^8 motif to F^5QQL^8 significantly reduced the cell surface levels of btGLUT4 to levels comparable to those of okGLUT4 or the mammalian GLUT4. These results indicate that specific amino acid motifs as well as the folding of the molecule appear to be important for the intracellular domains of the GLUT4 molecule to interact with the different regulatory proteins for proper traffic and specific compartment localization and/or retention.

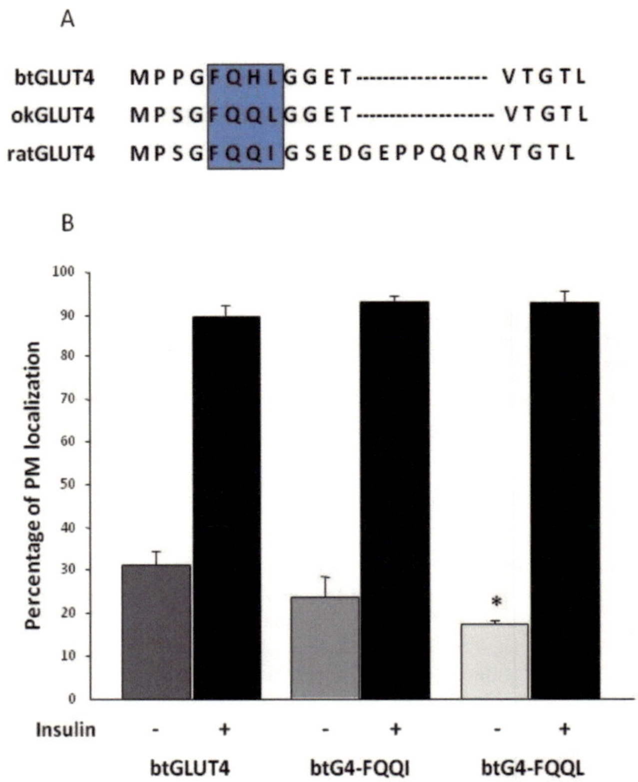

Figure 8. The elevated basal cell surface levels of btGLUT4 are reduced by mutating the F^5QHL^8 motif. (A) Amino acid sequence alignment of the N-terminal region of rat, brown trout (btGLUT4, AF247395) and coho salmon (okGLUT4, AF502957) GLUT4 molecules. The box encloses the important trafficking motif F^5QQI^8 partially conserved in the fish species. (B) Differentiated 3T3-L1 adipocytes expressing either btGLUT4 or any of the two point mutants (btGLUT4-FQQI or btGLUT4-FQQL) were incubated with or without insulin (100 nM, 30 min). Data is presented as percentage (mean ± SEM) of cells showing a complete plasma membrane (PM) rim obtained by counting 100 cells per condition in 3 independent experiments. Statistical analysis was performed by unpaired t-test against the wild type btGLUT4 at basal or insulin-stimulated conditions respectively (* denotes significance at $p < 0.05$).

An earlier study in mammals using chimeras between GLUT4 and Glut1 demonstrated that substituting the N-terminus and the intracellular loop of Glut1 for those of GLUT4 is sufficient to confer to the chimeric Glut1 protein the characteristics of GLUT4 in 3T3-L1 adipocytes [89]. Thus, in order to identify the protein domains in trout GLUT4 that confer its particular traffic characteristics (i.e. lower intracellular retention; higher PM levels under basal conditions), chimeric proteins were created that have the N-terminus (btN) or the intracellular loop (btL) of btGLUT4 in a rat GLUT4 backbone and were named btN-GLUT4 or btL-GLUT4, respectively. These constructs were then stably expressed in 3T3-L1 cells and their capacity to be retained in the cytosol under basal conditions and to respond to insulin were analyzed (Simoes, Planas and Camps, unpublished results). The results obtained indicated that all constructs were able to translocate to the PM in response to insulin but with certain differences among them (Figure 9). First, the insulin-stimulated translocation of btGLUT4 was lower than that of rat GLUT4. Second, btN-GLUT4 had the weakest response to insulin, suggesting a role for the N-terminus in the correct targeting of GLUT4 to the IRC or in the translocation of GLUT4 to the PM. Third, the substitution of the cytoplasmic loop in btL-GLUT4 caused a reduction in the response of rat GLUT4 to insulin comparable to that of btGLUT4. These preliminary results support the idea that the N-terminus and the cytoplasmic loop of GLUT4 are responsible for some of the trafficking differences between btGLUT4 and rat GLUT4.

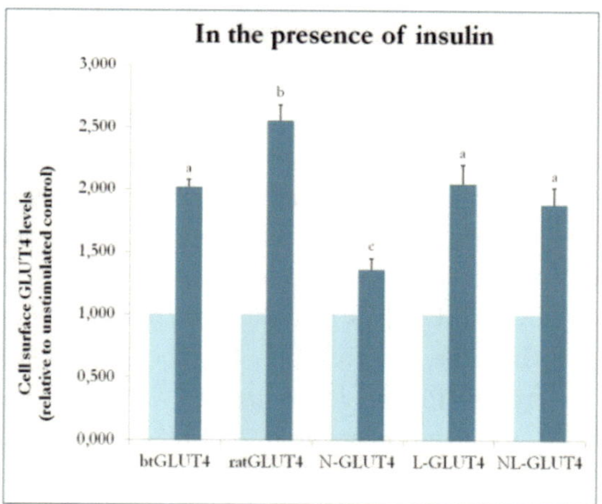

Figure 9. Cell surface levels of various GLUT4 constructs in the presence of insulin. N-GLUT4 and L-GLUT4 represent constructs with the amino terminus (N) or the intracellular loop (L) of btGLUT4 in a rat GLUT4 backbone, respectively. Differentiated 3T3-L1 adipocytes expressing the various GLUT4 constructs were incubated in the absence or presence of insulin (100nM) for 30 min and the determination of surface GLUT4 levels was performed as described in [32]. Cell surface GLUT4 is expressed relative to the unstimulated control for each cell line. Different letters indicate statistically significant differences ($p < 0.05$).

Following insulin stimulation, mammalian GLUT4 traffics and fuses with the PM, increasing its presence in the cell surface up to 10-fold; thus, supporting the increase in glucose uptake observed after feeding. Insulin increases the number of transporters at the PM not only by enhancing exocytosis but also by decreasing the rate of endocytosis [90-92]. Insulin exerts its effects through two different intracellular signaling pathways [15,93]. The first is the well-known pathway of phosphatidylinositol-3-kinase (PI3K)/protein kinase B (PKB), also known as Akt, that is necessary for GLUT4 translocation to occur [94,95] but not sufficient [96]. The second pathway is that including the Cbl associated protein (CAP), which binds the insulin receptor and activates a small GTPase from the Rho family named TC10, and that was described in adipocytes [97]. However, the TC10 pathway appears not to be involved in muscle cells, in which another Akt-independent input was shown to contribute to the cytoskeleton remodeling required for complete GLUT4 translocation [98,99]. Downstream of Akt, a protein named Akt substrate of 160 KDa (AS160) or TCB1D4, has been found to be the key to communicate the phosphorylation cascade initiated by insulin with the vesicle trafficking machinery [100,101]. AS160 has 6 residues of threonine/serine that can be phosphorylated to inhibit its activity, and contains a GTPase-activating protein (GAP) domain that in the basal state inactivates a series of Rab proteins, small GTPases from the Ras superfamily responsible of membrane trafficking [100]. Phosphorylation of AS160 by Akt inhibits its GAP activity, allowing the activation of the Rab proteins; thus, causing the translocation of GLUT4 to the PM [101,102]. The Rab members identified as responsible for GLUT4 trafficking in mammals are Rab8a, Rab10 and Rab14 [103-106]. In addition to regulating the movement of GLUT4 vesicles, AS160 has been demonstrated to be required for fully retaining GLUT4 into the IRC [107]. To demonstrate that AS160 phosphorylation is critical for GLUT4 translocation in mammals, a dominant-inhibitory form of AS160 was created by mutating 4 of its 6 phosphorylation sites (AS160-4P) [101]. When co-expressed in a cellular system together with rat GLUT4, the translocation of this molecule to the PM was blocked, as well as the increase in glucose uptake observed after insulin incubation [40,108]. Regarding their sensitivity towards AS160-4P, clear differences were observed between okGLUT4 and btGLUT4, with the former showing similar properties as those of mammalian GLUT4, and the latter being unaffected [79]. These results were in agreement with the differences observed between the two fish GLUT4 proteins in terms of their intracellular retention and support the hypothesis that AS160 may sequester okGLUT4, but not btGLUT4, in the IRC and that btGLUT4 may be more widely distributed inside the cell than the other GLUT4 transporters. Moreover, since the results obtained for btGLUT4 towards AS160 sensitivity agreed with those reported previously for a GLUT4-F5A mutant [40,73], the faster exocytic rate of btGLUT4 was suggested to be due to the lack of a conserved FQQI motif [32,79].

In summary, by investigating the trafficking characteristics of the two fish GLUT4 proteins (btGLUT4 and okGLUT4) compared with mammalian GLUT4 and Glut1, it is clear that important differences exist between these transporters (Figure 7). In this regard, okGLUT4 behaves in many aspects similarly to mammalian GLUT4 due to its sensitivity towards GGA and AS160; thus, supporting a role for these molecules in the regulation of the traffic of okGLUT4 synthesized *de novo* from the TGN into the IRC, and from the TGN into the PM in response to insulin, respectively. In contrast, btGLUT4 appears to be less regulated, trafficking to the IRC independently of GGA, as well as being retained in the IRC and exiting to the PM only in part under the control of AS160; therefore, moving towards the cell surface possibly, in part, through a constitutive pathway as that used by Glut1.

http://dx.doi.org/10.5772/58094

7. Conclusions and perspectives

All the evidence accumulated to date on the function and regulation of GLUT4 in fish indicates that the various molecular and cellular mechanisms regulating the amount of GLUT4 that is present at the cell surface in skeletal muscle and adipose tissue cells and that determine the amount of glucose uptake have been relatively well conserved during evolution from fish to mammals. Importantly, GLUT4 in fish is regulated by insulin at the level of mRNA and total protein amount as well as at the level of its abundance at the PM. In fish, like in mammals, GLUT4 responds to the effects of insulin by facilitating the uptake of glucose in insulin-sensitive tissues such as skeletal muscle. Therefore, GLUT4 plays an important role in mediating the hypoglycemic effects of insulin from fish to mammals and underscores the importance of the maintenance of glucose homeostasis, and the role of GLUT4 in this process, throughout vertebrates. However, the presence of a seemingly well conserved insulin-regulated mechanism of glucose transport involving GLUT4 contrasts with the relative glucose intolerance of teleost fish, that is evidenced by the lower ability of fish to clear a glucose load, when compared to mammals. It was initially hypothesized that the persistent hyperglycemia in fish may have been due to the possible lack of an insulin-regulated GLUT [25], given that fish have functional insulin receptors [109] and insulin is involved in the postprandial regulation of blood glucose levels [24]. The demonstration of the participation of an insulin-regulatable glucose transport system involving GLUT4 in skeletal muscle and adipose tissue of fish [26,31-32,59-60,70,79] rules out that fish may experience peripheral resistance to insulin. What today appears as a likely contribution to explain the poor regulation of glucose plasma levels in fish, when compared to mammals, are the particular transport characteristics and intracellular trafficking behavior of fish GLUT4. Functionally, fish GLUT4 differs from mammalian GLUT4 in that it has a lower affinity for glucose and a wider substrate specificity. In addition, the intracellular traffic of fish GLUT4 is somewhat different than that of mammalian GLUT4. Although insulin stimulates the translocation of fish GLUT4 to the PM, the intracellular route(s) used by fish GLUT4 to reach the PM are not as dependent on proteins required for the intracellular sorting and retention of mammalian GLUT4, which leads to the proportionally higher levels of fish GLUT4 at the PM under basal conditions. Differences in the intracellular traffic behavior of fish GLUT4, when compared to mammalian GLUT4, are likely due to differences in key protein motifs in GLUT4. Therefore, we propose that during evolution from fish to mammals, the control of glucose homeostasis has improved possibly due to the increase in the affinity of GLUT4 for glucose and to the improvement of the intracellular sorting and retention mechanisms of GLUT4 in insulin-sensitive cells.

Interestingly, GLUT4 from different fish species that contain slightly different amino acid sequences in key trafficking motifs can be considered natural mutants of mammalian GLUT4 and used to identify and further characterize amino acid motifs or protein domains in mammalian GLUT4 that are important for the regulation of the traffic of mammalian GLUT4. Our studies on the traffic behavior of chimeric GLUT4 proteins incorporating fish GLUT4 protein motifs into a mammalian GLUT4 backbone represent a first step in that direction. Given that the traffic of GLUT4 is dependent on the binding of GLUT4 to sorting and trafficking proteins that are not fully characterized in mammals, studies comparing the traffic of fish and mammalian GLUT4 could potentially identify important binding partners of mammalian GLUT4 that do not interact or interact poorly with fish GLUT4 motifs. Consequently, the comparative study of GLUT4 from evolutionarily distant species could contribute to our understanding of the biology of GLUT4 in health and disease.

Acknowledgements

Most of the work of the Planas laboratory described here has been supported by grants AGL2002-03987, AGL2005-01230, CSD2007-0002 and AGL2009-07006 to JVP from the Spanish Ministry of Science and Education. The authors would like to particularly thank Dr. Amira Klip (Hospital for Sick Children, University of Toronto) and Dr. Jeffrey Pessin (Albert Einstein College of Medicine, New York) for their stimulating collaborations and interest in the comparative aspects of GLUT4 biology.

Author details

Rubén Marín-Juez[1,3], Encarnación Capilla[1], Francisco Carvalho-Simoes[2,3], Marta Camps[2,3] and Josep V. Planas[1,3*]

*Address all correspondence to: jplanas@ub.edu

1 Departament de Fisiologia i Immunologia, Facultat de Biologia, Universitat de Barcelona, Spain

2 Departament de Biologia Molecular, Facultat de Biologia, Universitat de Barcelona, Spain

3 Institut de Biomedicina de la Universitat de Barcelona (IBUB), Barcelona, Spain

References

[1] James DE, Brown R, Navarro J, Pilch PF. Insulin-regulatable tissues express a unique insulin-sensitive glucose transport protein. Nature. 1988;333(6169):183–5.

[2] Fukumoto H, Kayano T, Buse JB, Edwards Y, Pilch PF, Bell GI, et al. Cloning and characterization of the major insulin-responsive glucose transporter expressed in human skeletal muscle and other insulin-responsive tissues. J Biol Chem. 1989;264(14): 7776–9.

[3] Birnbaum MJ. Identification of a novel gene encoding an insulin-responsive glucose transporter protein. Cell. 1989;57(2):305–15.

[4] Charron MJ, Brosius FC3, Alper SL, Lodish HF. A glucose transport protein expressed predominately in insulin-responsive tissues. Proc Natl Acad Sci USA. 1989;86(8):2535–9.

[5] Kaestner KH, Christy RJ, McLenithan JC, Braiterman LT, Cornelius P, Pekala PH, et al. Sequence, tissue distribution, and differential expression of mRNA for a putative insulin-responsive glucose transporter in mouse 3T3-L1 adipocytes. Proc Natl Acad Sci USA. 1989;86(9):3150–4.

[6] Huang S, Czech MP. The GLUT4 glucose transporter. Cell Metab. 2007;5(4):237–52.

[7] Keller K, Strube M, Mueckler M. Functional expression of the human HepG2 and rat adipocyte glucose transporters in Xenopus oocytes. Comparison of kinetic parameters. J Biol Chem. 1989;264(32):18884–9.

[8] Burant CF, Bell GI. Mammalian facilitative glucose transporters: evidence for similar substrate recognition sites in functionally monomeric proteins. Biochemistry. 1992;31(42):10414–20.

[9] Rumsey SC, Daruwala R, Al-Hasani H, Zarnowski MJ, Simpson IA, Levine M. Dehydroascorbic acid transport by GLUT4 in Xenopus oocytes and isolated rat adipocytes. J Biol Chem. 2000;275(36):28246–53.

[10] Uldry M, Ibberson M, Hosokawa M, Thorens B. GLUT2 is a high affinity glucosamine transporter. FEBS Lett. 2002;524(1-3):199–203.

[11] Mueckler M. Facilitative glucose transporters. Eur J Biochem. 1994;219(3):713–25.

[12] Rayner DV, Thomas ME, Trayhurn P. Glucose transporters (GLUTs 1-4) and their mRNAs in regions of the rat brain: insulin-sensitive transporter expression in the cerebellum. Can J Physiol Pharmacol. 1994;72(5):476–9.

[13] Shepherd PR, Kahn BB. Glucose transporters and insulin action--implications for insulin resistance and diabetes mellitus. N Engl J Med. 1999;341(4):248–57.

[14] Saltiel AR, Pessin JE. Insulin signaling pathways in time and space. Trends Cell Biol. 2002;12(2):65–71.

[15] Bryant NJ, Govers R, James DE. Regulated transport of the glucose transporter GLUT4. Nat Rev Mol Cell Biol. 2002;3(4):267–77.

[16] Kusari J, Verma US, Buse JB, Henry RR, Olefsky JM. Analysis of the gene sequences of the insulin receptor and the insulin-sensitive glucose transporter (GLUT-4) in patients with common-type non-insulin-dependent diabetes mellitus. J Clin Invest. 1991;88(4):1323–30.

[17] Friedel S, Antwerpen B, Hoch A, Vogel C, Grassl W, Geller F, et al. Glucose transporter 4 gene: association studies pertaining to alleles of two polymorphisms in extremely obese children and adolescents and in normal and underweight controls. Ann N Y Acad Sci. 2002;967:554–7.

[18] Karnieli E, Armoni M. Transcriptional regulation of the insulin-responsive glucose transporter GLUT4 gene: from physiology to pathology. Am J Physiol Endocrinol Metab. 2008;295(1):E38–45.

[19] Wood IS, Trayhurn P. Glucose transporters (GLUT and SGLT): expanded families of sugar transport proteins. Br J Nutr. 2003;89(1):3–9.

[20] Polakof S, Mommsen TP, Soengas JL. Glucosensing and glucose homeostasis: from fish to mammals. Comp Biochem Physiol B Mol Biol 2011;160:123-149.

[21] Moon TW. Glucose intolerance in teleost fish: fact or fiction? Comp Biochem Physiol B Biochem Mol Biol. 2001;129(2-3):243–9.

[22] Cowey JY, Walton MJ. Intermediary metabolism. In: Halver JE, editor. Fish Nutrition. 2nd ed. Sant Diego: Academic Press; 1989. pp. 259–329.

[23] Blasco J, FernandezBorras J, Marimon I, Requena A. Plasma glucose kinetics and tissue uptake in brown trout in vivo: Effect of an intravascular glucose load. J Comp Physiol B. 1996;165(7):534–41.

[24] Mommsen TP, Plisetskaya EM. Insulin in Fishes and Agnathans-History, Structure, and Metabolic-Regulation. Rev Aquat Sci. 1991;4(2-3):225–59.

[25] Wright JRJ, O'Hali W, Yang H, Han XX, Bonen A. GLUT-4 Deficiency and severe peripheral resistance to insulin in the teleost fish tilapia. Gen Comp Endocrinol. 1998;111(1):20–7.

[26] Planas JV, Capilla E, Gutiérrez J. Molecular identification of a glucose transporter from fish muscle. FEBS Lett. 2000;481(3):266–70.

[27] Welch KC, Allalou A, Sehgal P, Cheng J, Ashok A. Glucose Transporter Expression in an Avian Nectarivore: The Ruby-Throated Hummingbird (Archilochus colubris). PLoS ONE. 2013;8(10):e77003.

[28] Louis A, Muffato M, Roest Crollius H. Genomicus: five genome browsers for comparative genomics in eukaryota. Nucleic Acids Res. 2013;41:D700-705.

[29] Zorzano A, Palacín M, Gumà A. Mechanisms regulating GLUT4 glucose transporter expression and glucose transport in skeletal muscle. Acta Physiol Scand. 2005;183(1): 43–58.

[30] Marín-Juez R, Díaz M, Morata J, Planas JV. Mechanisms Regulating GLUT4 Transcription in Skeletal Muscle Cells Are Highly Conserved across Vertebrates. PLoS ONE. 2013;8(11):e80628.

[31] Capilla E, Díaz M, Albalat A, Navarro I, Pessin JE, Keller K, et al. Functional characterization of an insulin-responsive glucose transporter (GLUT4) from fish adipose tissue. Am J Physiol Endocrinol Metab. 2004;287(2):E348–57.

[32] Díaz M, Antonescu CN, Capilla E, Klip A, Planas JV. Fish glucose transporter (GLUT)-4 differs from rat GLUT4 in its traffic characteristics but can translocate to

the cell surface in response to insulin in skeletal muscle cells. Endocrinology. 2007;148(11):5248–57.

[33] Seatter MJ, la Rue De SA, Porter LM, Gould GW. QLS motif in transmembrane helix VII of the glucose transporter family interacts with the C-1 position of D-glucose and is involved in substrate selection at the exofacial binding site. Biochemistry. 1998;37(5):1322–6.

[34] Wellner M, Monden I, Keller K. From triple cysteine mutants to the cysteine-less glucose transporter GLUT1: a functional analysis. FEBS Lett. 1995;370(1-2):19–22.

[35] Doege H, Schurmann A, Ohnimus H, Monser V, Holman GD, Joost HG. Serine-294 and threonine-295 in the exofacial loop domain between helices 7 and 8 of glucose transporters (GLUT) are involved in the conformational alterations during the transport process. Biochem J. 1998;329 (Pt 2):289–93.

[36] Garippa RJ, Judge TW, James DE, McGraw TE. The amino terminus of GLUT4 functions as an internalization motif but not an intracellular retention signal when substituted for the transferrin receptor cytoplasmic domain. J Cell Biol. 1994;124(5):705–15.

[37] Blot V, McGraw TE. Molecular mechanisms controlling GLUT4 intracellular retention. Mol Biol Cell. 2008;19(8):3477–87.

[38] Martinez-Arca S, Lalioti VS, Sandoval IV. Intracellular targeting and retention of the glucose transporter GLUT4 by the perinuclear storage compartment involves distinct carboxyl-tail motifs. J Cell Sci. 2000;113 (Pt 10):1705–15.

[39] Pessin JE, Thurmond DC, Elmendorf JS, Coker KJ, Okada S. Molecular basis of insulin-stimulated GLUT4 vesicle trafficking. Location! Location! Location! J Biol Chem. 1999;274(5):2593–6.

[40] Capilla E, Suzuki N, Pessin JE, Hou JC. The glucose transporter 4 FQQI motif is necessary for Akt substrate of 160-kilodalton-dependent plasma membrane translocation but not Golgi-localized (gamma)-ear-containing Arf-binding protein-dependent entry into the insulin-responsive storage compartment. Mol Endocrinol. 2007;21(12): 3087–99.

[41] Al-Hasani H, Kunamneni RK, Dawson K, Hinck CS, Müller-Wieland D, Cushman SW. Roles of the N-and C-termini of GLUT4 in endocytosis. J Cell Sci. 2002;115(Pt 1): 131–40.

[42] Gould GW, Lienhard GE. Expression of a functional glucose transporter in Xenopus oocytes. Biochemistry. 1989;28(24):9447–52.

[43] Gould GW, Thomas HM, Jess TJ, Bell GI. Expression of human glucose transporters in Xenopus oocytes: kinetic characterization and substrate specificities of the erythrocyte, liver, and brain isoforms. Biochemistry. 1991;30(21):5139–45.

[44] Nishimura H, Pallardo FV, Seidner GA, Vannucci S, Simpson IA, Birnbaum MJ. Kinetics of GLUT1 and GLUT4 glucose transporters expressed in Xenopus oocytes. J Biol Chem. 1993;268(12):8514–20.

[45] Teerijoki H, Krasnov A, Pitkanen TI, Mölsä H. Cloning and characterization of glucose transporter in teleost fish rainbow trout (Oncorhynchus mykiss). Biochim Biophys Acta. 2000;1494(3):290–4.

[46] Soengas J, Moon T. Uptake and metabolism of glucose, alanine and lactate by red blood cells of the American eel Anguilla rostrata. J Exp Biol. 1995;198(Pt 4):877–88.

[47] Basketter DA, Widdas WF. Competitive inhibition of hexose transfer in human erythrocytes by Cytochalasin B. J Physiol. 1977;265(1):39P–40P.

[48] Basketter DA, Widdas WF. Asymmetry of the hexose transfer system in human erythrocytes. Comparison of the effects of cytochalasin B, phloretin and maltose as competitive inhibitors. J Physiol. 1978;278:389–401.

[49] Deves R, Krupka RM. Cytochalasin B and the kinetics of inhibition of biological transport: a case of asymmetric binding to the glucose carrier. Biochim Biophys Acta. 1978;510(2):339–48.

[50] Tiihonen K, Nikinmaa M, Lappivaara J. Glucose transport in carp erythrocytes: individual variation and effects of osmotic swelling, extracellular pH and catecholamines. J Exp Biol. 1995;198(Pt 2):577–83.

[51] Tse CM, Young JD. Glucose transport in fish erythrocytes: variable cytochalasin-B-sensitive hexose transport activity in the common eel (Anguilla japonica) and transport deficiency in the paddyfield eel (Monopterus albus) and rainbow trout (Salmo gairdneri). J Exp Biol. 1990;148:367–83.

[52] Young JD, Yao SYM, Tse CM, Davies A, Baldwin SA. Functional and Molecular Characteristics of a Primitive Vertebrate Glucose-Transporter-Studies of Glucose-Transport by Erythrocytes from the Pacific Hagfish (Eptatretus-Stouti). J Exp Biol. 1994;186:23–41.

[53] Murata H, Hruz PW, Mueckler M. The mechanism of insulin resistance caused by HIV protease inhibitor therapy. J Biol Chem. 2000;275(27):20251–4.

[54] Murata H, Hruz PW, Mueckler M. Indinavir inhibits the glucose transporter isoform GLUT4 at physiologic concentrations. AIDS (London, England). 2002;16(6):859–63.

[55] Rudich A, Klip A. Push/pull mechanisms of GLUT4 traffic in muscle cells. Acta Physiol Scand. 2003;178(4):297–308.

[56] Hall JR, Short CE, Driedzic WR. Sequence of Atlantic cod (Gadus morhua) GLUT4, GLUT2 and GPDH: Developmental stage expression, tissue expression and relationship to starvation-induced changes in blood glucose. J Exp Biol. 2006;209(Pt 22):4490–502.

[57] Panserat S, Skiba-Cassy S, Seiliez I, Lansard M, Plagnes-Juan E, Vachot C, et al. Metformin improves postprandial glucose homeostasis in rainbow trout fed dietary carbohydrates: a link with the induction of hepatic lipogenic capacities? Am J Physiol Regul Integr Comp Physiol. 2009;297(3):R707–15.

[58] McGowan KM, Long SD, Pekala PH. Glucose transporter gene expression: regulation of transcription and mRNA stability. Pharmac Ther. 1995;66(3):465–505.

[59] Díaz M, Vraskou Y, Gutiérrez J, Planas JV. Expression of rainbow trout glucose transporters GLUT1 and GLUT4 during in vitro muscle cell differentiation and regulation by insulin and IGF-I. Am J Physiol Regul Integr Comp Physiol. 2009;296(3):R794–800.

[60] Capilla E, Díaz M, Gutiérrez J, Planas JV. Physiological regulation of the expression of a GLUT4 homolog in fish skeletal muscle. Am J Physiol Endocrinol Metab. 2002;283(1):E44–9.

[61] Neufer PD, Carey JO, Dohm GL. Transcriptional regulation of the gene for glucose transporter GLUT4 in skeletal muscle. Effects of diabetes and fasting. J Biol Chem. 1993;268(19):13824–9.

[62] MacLean PS, Zheng D, Jones JP, Olson AL, Dohm GL. Exercise-induced transcription of the muscle glucose transporter (GLUT 4) gene. Biochem Biophys Res Comm. 2002;292(2):409–14.

[63] Jorgensen SB, Richter EA, Wojtaszewski JFP. Role of AMPK in skeletal muscle metabolic regulation and adaptation in relation to exercise. J Physiol. 2006;574(Pt 1):17–31.

[64] Felip O, Ibarz A, Fernández-Borràs J, Beltrán M, Martín-Pérez M, Planas JV, et al. Tracing metabolic routes of dietary carbohydrate and protein in rainbow trout (Oncorhynchus mykiss) using stable isotopes ([^{13}C]starch and [^{15}N]protein): effects of gelatinisation of starches and sustained swimming. Br J Nutr. 2012;107(6):834–44.

[65] Magnoni LJ, Crespo D, Ibarz A, Blasco J, Fernández-Borràs J, Planas JV. Effects of sustained swimming on the red and white muscle transcriptome of rainbow trout (Oncorhynchus mykiss) fed a carbohydrate-rich diet. Comp Biochem Physiol A Mol Integr Physiol. 2013;166(3):1–12.

[66] Magnoni LJ, Vraskou Y, Palstra AP, Planas JV. AMP-activated protein kinase plays an important evolutionary conserved role in the regulation of glucose metabolism in fish skeletal muscle cells. PLoS ONE. 2012;7(2):e31219.

[67] Girón MD, Sevillano N, Vargas AM, Domínguez J, Guinovart JJ, Salto R. The glucose-lowering agent sodium tungstate increases the levels and translocation of GLUT4 in L6 myotubes through a mechanism associated with ERK1/2 and MEF2D. Diabetologia. 2008;51(7):1285–95.

[68] Cooke DW, Lane MD. The transcription factor nuclear factor I mediates repression of the GLUT4 promoter by insulin. J Biol Chem. 1999;274(18):12917–24.

[69] Hallakou S, Doare L, Foufelle F, Kergoat M, Guerre-Millo M, Berthault MF, et al. Pioglitazone induces in vivo adipocyte differentiation in the obese Zucker fa/fa rat. Diabetes. 1997;46(9):1393–9.

[70] Díaz M, Capilla E, Planas JV. Physiological regulation of glucose transporter (GLUT4) protein content in brown trout (Salmo trutta) skeletal muscle. J Exp Biol. 2007;210(Pt 13):2346–51.

[71] Dugani CB, Klip A. Glucose transporter 4: cycling, compartments and controversies. EMBO reports. 2005;6(12):1137-42.

[72] Vraskou Y, Roher N, Díaz M, Antonescu CN, Mackenzie SA, Planas JV. Direct involvement of tumor necrosis factor-α in the regulation of glucose uptake in rainbow trout muscle cells. Am J Physiol Regul Integr Comp Physiol. 2011;300(3):R716–23.

[73] Watson RT, Kanzaki M, Pessin JE. Regulated membrane trafficking of the insulin-responsive glucose transporter 4 in adipocytes. Endocr Rev. 2004;25(2):177–204.

[74] Karylowski O, Zeigerer A, Cohen A, McGraw TE. GLUT4 is retained by an intracellular cycle of vesicle formation and fusion with endosomes. Mol Biol Cell. 2004;15(2): 870–82.

[75] Shewan AM, van Dam EM, Martin S, Luen TB, Hong W, Bryant NJ, et al. GLUT4 recycles via a trans-Golgi network (TGN) subdomain enriched in Syntaxins 6 and 16 but not TGN38: involvement of an acidic targeting motif. Mol Biol Cell. 2003;14(3): 973–86.

[76] Malide D, Dwyer NK, Blanchette-Mackie EJ, Cushman SW. Immunocytochemical evidence that GLUT4 resides in a specialized translocation post-endosomal VAMP2-positive compartment in rat adipose cells in the absence of insulin. J Histochem Cytochem. 1997;45(8):1083–96.

[77] Martin OJ, Lee A, McGraw TE. GLUT4 distribution between the plasma membrane and the intracellular compartments is maintained by an insulin-modulated bipartite dynamic mechanism. J Biol Chem. 2006;281(1):484–90.

[78] Satoh S, Nishimura H, Clark AE, Kozka IJ, Vannucci SJ, Simpson IA, et al. Use of bismannose photolabel to elucidate insulin-regulated GLUT4 subcellular trafficking kinetics in rat adipose cells. Evidence that exocytosis is a critical site of hormone action. J Biol Chem. 1993;268(24):17820–9.

[79] Capilla E, Díaz M, Hou JC, Planas JV, Pessin JE. High basal cell surface levels of fish GLUT4 are related to reduced sensitivity of insulin-induced translocation toward GGA and AS160 inhibition in adipocytes. Am J Physiol Endocrinol Metab. 2010;298(2):E329–36.

[80] Slot JW, Geuze HJ, Gigengack S, Lienhard GE, James DE. Immuno-localization of the insulin regulatable glucose transporter in brown adipose tissue of the rat. J Cell Biol. 1991;113(1):123–35.

[81] Li LV, Kandror KV. Golgi-localized, gamma-ear-containing, Arf-binding protein adaptors mediate insulin-responsive trafficking of glucose transporter 4 in 3T3-L1 adipocytes. Mol Endocrinol. 2005;19(8):2145–53.

[82] Shi J, Kandror KV. Sortilin is essential and sufficient for the formation of GLUT4 storage vesicles in 3T3-L1 adipocytes. Dev Cell. 2005;9(1):99–108.

[83] Jordens I, Molle D, Xiong W, Keller SR, McGraw TE. Insulin-regulated aminopeptidase is a key regulator of GLUT4 trafficking by controlling the sorting of GLUT4 from endosomes to specialized insulin-regulated vesicles. Mol Biol Cell. 2010;21(12): 2034–44.

[84] Yu C, Cresswell J, Löffler MG, Bogan JS. The glucose transporter 4-regulating protein TUG is essential for highly insulin-responsive glucose uptake in 3T3-L1 adipocytes. J Biol Chem. 2007;282(10):7710–22.

[85] Khan AH, Capilla E, Hou JC, Watson RT, Smith JR, Pessin JE. Entry of newly synthesized GLUT4 into the insulin-responsive storage compartment is dependent upon both the amino terminus and the large cytoplasmic loop. J Biol Chem. 2004;279(36): 37505–11.

[86] Piper RC, Tai C, Kulesza P, Pang S, Warnock D, Baenziger J, et al. GLUT-4 NH2 terminus contains a phenylalanine-based targeting motif that regulates intracellular sequestration. J Cell Biol. 1993;121(6):1221–32.

[87] Piper RC, Tai C, Slot JW, Hahn CS, Rice CM, Huang H, et al. The efficient intracellular sequestration of the insulin-regulatable glucose transporter (GLUT-4) is conferred by the NH2 terminus. J Cell Biol. 1992;117(4):729–43.

[88] Melvin DR, Marsh BJ, Walmsley AR, James DE, Gould GW. Analysis of amino and carboxy terminal GLUT-4 targeting motifs in 3T3-L1 adipocytes using an endosomal ablation technique. Biochemistry. 1999;38(5):1456–62.

[89] Khan AH, Capilla E, Hou JC, Watson RT, Smith JR, Pessin JE. Entry of newly synthesized GLUT4 into the insulin-responsive storage compartment is dependent upon both the amino terminus and the large cytoplasmic loop. J Biol Chem. 2004;279(36): 37505–11.

[90] Ceresa BP, Kao AW, Santeler SR, Pessin JE. Inhibition of clathrin-mediated endocytosis selectively attenuates specific insulin receptor signal transduction pathways. Mol Cel Biol. 1998;18(7):3862–70.

[91] Kao AW, Ceresa BP, Santeler SR, Pessin JE. Expression of a dominant interfering dynamin mutant in 3T3L1 adipocytes inhibits GLUT4 endocytosis without affecting insulin signaling. J Biol Chem. 1998;273(39):25450–7.

[92] Shibata H, Suzuki Y, Omata W, Tanaka S, Kojima I. Dissection of GLUT4 recycling pathway into exocytosis and endocytosis in rat adipocytes. Evidence that GTP-binding proteins are involved in both processes. J Biol Chem. 1995;270(19):11489–95.

[93] Hou JC, Pessin JE. Ins (endocytosis) and outs (exocytosis) of GLUT4 trafficking. Curr Opin Cell Biol. 2007;19(4):466–73.

[94] Yang J, Clarke JF, Ester CJ, Young PW, Kasuga M, Holman GD. Phosphatidylinositol 3-kinase acts at an intracellular membrane site to enhance GLUT4 exocytosis in 3T3-L1 cells. Biochem J. 1996;313 (Pt 1):125–31.

[95] Shepherd PR, Withers DJ, Siddle K. Phosphoinositide 3-kinase: the key switch mechanism in insulin signalling. Biochem J. 1998;333 (Pt 3):471–90.

[96] Czech MP, Corvera S. Signaling mechanisms that regulate glucose transport. J Biol Chem. 1999;274(4):1865–8.

[97] Baumann CA, Ribon V, Kanzaki M, Thurmond DC, Mora S, Shigematsu S, et al. CAP defines a second signalling pathway required for insulin-stimulated glucose transport. Nature. 2000;407(6801):202–7.

[98] JeBailey L, Rudich A, Huang X, Di Ciano-Oliveira C, Kapus A, Klip A. Skeletal muscle cells and adipocytes differ in their reliance on TC10 and Rac for insulin-induced actin remodeling. Mol Endocrinol. 2004;18(2):359–72.

[99] Patel N, Rudich A, Khayat ZA, Garg R, Klip A. Intracellular segregation of phosphatidylinositol-3,4,5-trisphosphate by insulin-dependent actin remodeling in L6 skeletal muscle cells. Mol Cel Biol. 2003;23(13):4611–26.

[100] Kane S, Sano H, Liu SC, Asara JM, Lane WS, Garner CC, et al. A method to identify serine kinase substrates. Akt phosphorylates a novel adipocyte protein with a Rab GTPase-activating protein (GAP) domain. J Biol Chem. 2002;277(25):22115–8.

[101] Sano H, Kane S, Sano E, Miinea CP, Asara JM, Lane WS, et al. Insulin-stimulated phosphorylation of a Rab GTPase-activating protein regulates GLUT4 translocation. J Biol Chem. 2003;278(17):14599–602.

[102] Sakamoto K, Holman GD. Emerging role for AS160/TBC1D4 and TBC1D1 in the regulation of GLUT4 traffic. Am J Physiol Endocrinol Metab. 2008;295(1):E29–37.

[103] Ishikura S, Bilan PJ, Klip A. Rabs 8A and 14 are targets of the insulin-regulated Rab-GAP AS160 regulating GLUT4 traffic in muscle cells. Biochem Biophys Res Comm. 2007;353(4):1074–9.

[104] Ishikura S, Koshkina A, Klip A. Small G proteins in insulin action: Rab and Rho families at the crossroads of signal transduction and GLUT4 vesicle traffic. Acta Physiol (Oxf). 2008;192(1):61–74.

[105] Sano H, Eguez L, Teruel MN, Fukuda M, Chuang TD, Chavez JA, et al. Rab10, a target of the AS160 Rab GAP, is required for insulin-stimulated translocation of GLUT4 to the adipocyte plasma membrane. Cell Metab. 2007;5(4):293–303.

[106] Sadacca LA, Bruno J, Wen J, Xiong W, McGraw TE. Specialized sorting of GLUT4 and its recruitment to the cell surface are independently regulated by distinct Rabs. Mol Biol Cell. 2013;24(16):2544–57.

[107] Eguez L, Lee A, Chavez JA, Miinea CP, Kane S, Lienhard GE, et al. Full intracellular retention of GLUT4 requires AS160 Rab GTPase activating protein. Cell Metab. 2005;2(4):263–72.

[108] Zeigerer A, McBrayer MK, McGraw TE. Insulin stimulation of GLUT4 exocytosis, but not its inhibition of endocytosis, is dependent on RabGAP AS160. Mol Biol Cell. 2004;15(10):4406–15.

[109] Planas JV, Méndez E, Baños N, Capilla E, Castillo J, Navarro I, et al. Fish insulin, IGF-I and IGP-II receptors: A phylogenetic approach. Am Zool. 2000;40(2):223–33.

Section 2

Mechanisms of Glucose Homeostasis

Chapter 3

The Effects of Energy Intake, Insulin Therapy and Physical Activity on Glucose Homeostasis in Children and Adolescents with Type 1 Diabetes Mellitus

Aleksandra Żebrowska, Marcin Sikora,
Przemysława Jarosz-Chobot,
Barbara Głuchowska and Michał Plewa

Additional information is available at the end of the chapter

http://dx.doi.org/10.5772/57590

1. Introduction

Insulin therapy, dietary management, and physical activity constitute an essential element in prevention and treatment for children and adolescents with type 1 diabetes mellitus (T1DM). Regular physical activity positively affects metabolic and cardiovascular functions, and its benefits include enhanced insulin sensitivity, decreased fat mass, improved lipid profile and cardiovascular fitness [1-5]. All of these metabolic changes prevent the development of metabolic syndrome, decrease the risk of type 2 diabetes mellitus (T2DM), and are beneficial for patients with type 1 diabetes mellitus (T1DM) [6-12].

The classification of the American Diabetes Association defines four major forms of diabetes mellitus [13]. The major groups are: type 1 and type 2, gestational diabetes and diabetes due to other known causes. Type 1 diabetes mellitus is characterized by beta cell destruction caused by an autoimmune process, usually leading to absolute insulin deficiency [14-15]. Type 1 diabetes is also subdivided according to whether cell destruction is caused by the immune or other processes, and be classified as type1A or type 1B diabetes mellitus [13-14]. Type 1 diabetes, formerly known as juvenile-onset diabetes, accounts for 10-15 percent of all cases of diabetes mellitus. Approximately one-half of individuals develop the disease within the first two decades of life, making T1DM one of the most common chronic diseases of childhood. The reports of World Health Organization on the incidence of T1DM showed the greatest increase in the incidence rate among young children aged 4 to 9 years. Such high increase of incidence rate of type 1 diabetes mellitus suggests an epidemic tendency in many countries [17-18]. The fact that the incidence of type 1 diabetes mellitus is the highest among young population has increased the interest in the role of physical activity in the treatment of the disease [7, 16].

Insulin is a hormone produced by the pancreatic β cells. It is not only central to regulating carbohydrate, protein and fat metabolism, but also acts as a critical T1DM autoantigen. Autoimmune distraction of pancreatic β cells leads to insulin deficiency and consequent metabolic decomposition of glucose homeostasis [19-22].

Multidisciplinary research on the pathogenesis of T1DM indicates an involvement of genes predisposing to autoimmune damage to the pancreatic β cells [23-24]. It has been suggested that type 1 diabetes is a complex polygenic disease. The main susceptibility genes code for polymorphic HLA molecules and, in particular, alleles of class II MHC genes [15, 25]. Risk of T1DM progression is conferred by specific HLA DR/DQ alleles (e.g., DRB1*03-DQB1*0201 [DR3] or DRB1*04-DQB1*0302 [DR4]. The HLA alleles such as DQB1*0602 are associated with dominant protection against the disease [26]. Polymorphism of a variable nucleotide tandem repeat of the proinsulin gene and a single amino acid change of a gene termed PTPN22, a tyrosine phosphatase that influences T cell receptor signaling, are associated with increased risk for diabetes [15]. In physiological conditions there is balance between pathogenic T cells that mediate disease and regulatory cells that control autoimmunity. However, in T1DM, the balance between pathogenic and regulatory T cells is altered [27]. Thus, the ability to identify individuals at high risk for type 1 diabetes using genetic and/or autoantibody markers has been a main goal of the diabetes research and T1DM prediction strategies [20, 28].

Early diagnosis has expanded the chance for pharmacological treatments for diabetic children and adolescents. Autoimmune destruction of insulin-producing pancreatic β cells requires constant administration of various insulin preparations designed to meet basal and meal-dependent insulin requirements. In recent years, several new insulin analogs have been developed including short-acting insulin analogs with different pharmacokinetic properties [29-30]; the preparations have been recommended for tight control of blood glucose concentrations and significantly reduction of diabetic complications [31].

There is compelling evidence indicating that individuals who have been using intensive insulin therapy should participate in regular physical activity [1, 7, 32]. Findings from most experimental and questionnaire studies in youth suggest a positive relationship between physical activity and health benefits [33-35]. Regular physical activity in people with diabetes increases the capacity to maintain appropriate plasma glucose levels and enhances the patient's metabolic capacity during and after exercise [36-37]. However, in children and adolescents with type 1 diabetes, it may also be responsible for the occurrence of some adverse reactions such as hypoglycemia, hyperglycemia, ketosis and diabetes-related complications. These effects of exercise on glycemic control depend on several factors, such as starting levels of glycaemia, type, intensity of exercise, and the use of exogenous insulin and insulin secretagogues [38].

Contraction of skeletal muscle increases glucose metabolism through an insulin-independent pathway. In this mechanism, glucose delivery is facilitated by an increase in blood flow to the working muscle groups. Regular aerobic exercise increases the synthesis of glucose transporter (ie. GLUT 4) and enzymes to exercising muscles [39]. At rest, muscles mainly draw their energy from fats; hormonal control is a result of balance between insulin and glucagon secretion.

The metabolic adaptation during exercise is sequentially characteristic for each different phase of requirement of the exercising muscle. The first mechanism available for muscle contraction is to access energy from adenosine triphosphate (ATP) breakdown. Then, the high-energy phosphate from creatine phosphate (CP) is used to resynthesize ATP from adenosine diphosphate (ADP). The limited supplies of CP in the muscle require increased energy production from the non-oxidative (anaerobic) glycolytic pathway [40]. The fuel for this pathway is glucose from the blood or glucose stored in the muscle in the form of glycogen. The end product of glycolysis is pyruvic acid, which may be further processed to produce energy in the oxidative pathway or can be removed to form lactic acid or alanine. In muscle cell mitochondria, the oxidative pathway can use fats or lipids as a fuel. Both glucose, through the formation of pyruvic acid, and lipids are oxidized in the tricarboxylic acid (TCA) cycle (Krebs cycle) [41]. It is well documented that the ATP resynthesis depends on glucose transport into the cell [42-43]. One of the beneficial effects of exercise on glucose homeostasis in people with diabetes is a marked stimulation of blood glucose utilization via the insulin independent mechanism. Increased synthesis of GLUT-4 through insulin-independent pathway in the muscles results in the enhancement of the glycolytic and oxidative energy produced during exercise and post-exercise glycogen stores [44]. Increased glucose uptake is usually observed after a single bout of exercise even when insulin level decreases [45-46].

Muscle cells differ in their contractile and metabolic properties [47]. Their different recruitment depends on the exercise intensity and duration [48]. All the aforementioned processes allow describing the fuel mobilization and muscle metabolism at three levels of exercise intensity ie: low-, moderate-, and high-intensity exercise. During low-intensity exercise, energy for muscle contraction is supplied predominantly by oxidation of carbohydrates and free fatty acids (FFAs) mobilized from the adipose tissue and supplied by intramuscular triglycerides (TGs). The predominance of oxidative metabolism during low-intensity exercise is a consequence of selective recruitment of oxidative muscle fibers (type I). At moderate-intensity exercise, performed in the range of 50% to 75% of VO_{2max}, approximately half of the expended energy is derived from intramuscular lipids whereas the rest is derived from carbohydrates. Muscle glycogen and blood glucose contribute to carbohydrate utilization in 80 and 20%, respectively. Adipose tissue FFAs provide a bit more than half of the lipid fuel, and the rest is supplied by intramuscular TGs [49]. This pattern of fuel use is a consequence of the metabolic characteristics of the type IIa muscle fiber recruited during moderate-intensity exercise [50].

At high-intensity exercise (above 80% of VO_{2max}), about three quarters of total energy cost of exercise is supplied by glucose mainly derived from muscle glycogenolysis [36, 51]. FFA secretion is blocked by the vasoconstrictive action of catecholamine and increased concentration of lactic acid. High concentrations of lactate indirectly facilitate carbohydrate metabolism [52]. High concentrations of glycolytic enzymes activate ATP hydrolysis and anaerobic glycolysis [53]; type IIb glycolytic muscle fibers are preferentially recruited during high-intensity exercise [54-55].

It has been well documented that participation in low and moderate-intensity exercise by individuals with T1DM results in decreased blood glucose concentrations [6, 56-57]. In patients with diabetes, the effect of low-to-moderate intensity exercise varies according to the starting levels of glycaemia. In T1DM patients with pretraining hyperglycemia and ketosis resulting from insulin underdosing, a session of moderate-intensity exercise may increase hyperglycemia [36, 58]. In contrast, when patients with type 1 diabetes are treated with insulin and display mild to moderate hyperglycemia, exercise can lower plasma glucose concentrations thus preventing an episode of hypoglycemia [59-60].

The currently available data suggest that patients with T1DM are less likely to develop hypoglycemia during high-intensity exercise than when they engage in low-intensity exercise [57, 61]. There is evidence that high-intensity exercise added to low-or moderate-intensity exercise may maintain blood glucose levels within the normal physiological range and thus minimize the risk of hypoglycemia [62-63]. Guelfi et al. 2005 first demonstrated beneficial effects of the above mentioned exercise combinations on blood glucose levels. The effect is partly due to the fact that intermittent high-intensity exercise (defined as exercise involving repeated bouts of short duration), intense activity and alternating intervals of low-to moderate-intensity exercise are typical of many field sports and spontaneous physical activity in children and adolescents [36, 64-65].

The knowledge of the interactions between specific insulin preparations and various forms of exercise is essential to optimizing glycaemic control with minimizing the potential for derangements in glucose homeostasis [66]. The challenge in diabetic patients is to maintain glucose control during physical activity of varying intensity and to effectively decrease hyperglycemia as a result of lower catecholamine levels [67-68].

One of the most important therapeutic recommendations in type 1 diabetes is to lower the percentage of serum glycated hemoglobin, a long-term indicator of glycaemic status [69-70]. Glycated hemoglobin A_1c (HbA_1c) indicates the percentage of total hemoglobin that is bound by glucose and is formed in a non-enzymatic glycation pathway by hemoglobin's exposure to plasma glucose. International Expert Committee has recently recommended that HbA_1c might be a better means of diagnosing diabetes than measuring fasting and/or post-challenge glucose, and established HbA1c $\geq 6.5\%$ as the cut point for diagnosing the disease [69-73].

Type 1 diabetes is among the most common chronic conditions in childhood, occurring with increasing frequency, particularly in children aged five years or less [74]. Considering its complexity as well as invasive and continuous treatment, the disease can have a significant effect on children, parents and other family members by affecting many aspects of their lives. One of the beneficial effects of exercise on glucose homeostasis in people with diabetes is a marked stimulation of blood glucose utilization via the insulin independent mechanism. However, the effect of exercise on glycemic control in diabetes depends on several factors including exercise intensity, starting levels of glycaemia and use of exogenous insulin [75-77]. Therefore, the aim of the study was to investigate the effect of physical activity on glycaemic control in children and adolescents suffering from type 1 diabetes mellitus. Another study objective was to evaluate changes in glucose concentrations, glyceaemia, and glycated hemoglobin level in diabetic patients in response to regular exercise during diabetes camps.

http://dx.doi.org/10.5772/57590

2. Methods

2.1. Study participants

The study group comprised a total of 53 (27 girls and 26 boys) children and adolescents with type 1 diabetes mellitus (T1DM). Mean age was 11.8 ± 2.4 years (range 5 to 17 years); duration of diabetes was 2.8 ± 1.6 years (Table 1). All subjects lived and attended schools in Silesian Industrial Region in Poland and were recruited at the Diabetes Clinic of the Silesian Center for Child Health. They were treated with recombinant human insulin divided into daily doses, and performed self-monitoring of blood glucose on glycaemic control. The types of insulin used were: NovoRapid, Lantus, Humalog, Apidra. Only patients free of diabetic complications were enrolled. The other criteria for inclusion were no personal history of other cardiovascular or metabolic diseases, no simultaneous participation in another clinical trial, being free of any acute infections up to one week prior to the study, and HbA1c < 7.5%.

The medical history and information about diabetes etiology of the study participants were prepared by medical personnel. The adolescents and their parents were presented with a comprehensive description of the aim and methods of the study. Written consents were requested and obtained from all parents. The study protocol was approved by the Ethics Committee of the Academy of Physical Education in Katowice, Poland, and conformed to the standards set by the Declaration of Helsinki.

3. Measures

Height and body mass (mean ± SD) of the participants were measured according to standard procedures [78]. Body mass index (BMI) was calculated as weight (kg) divided by height (m) squared. All subjects were characterized by normal-weight according to international BMI cutoff values and BMI centiles [79] (Table 1).

The first group were monitored during their school classes (GrS; n=25). We assessed glycemia, diet and physical activity during the school day and leisure time. The other group comprised participants of a rehabilitation programme at a summer camp for diabetic children, organized by the Polish Society for Children and Youth with Diabetes. (GrR; n=28).

Physical activity (PA) assessment was performed using accelerometers (accelerometer ActiGraph GT3X+, USA). The first PA indicator was the number of steps per day (steps/day) while the other indicator was daily energy expenditure of physical activity (kcal/kg/day). According to recommendations, the children wore a device placed firmly on an elastic belt on the right hip. During the seven-day monitoring period, the accelerometers were taken off only at bedtime and before potential contact with water [33, 80-81]. The criteria of the 2001–2002 President's Challenge Physical Activity and Fitness Awards Program were used to assess physical activity [82]. The authors recommended that the daily number of steps, hops or position changes should be about 13,000 in boys and 11,000 in girls at least 5 days a week for a standard healthy base. Thus, the daily active energy expenditure should be at least 11 kcal/kg/day in boys and 9 kcal/kg/day in girls on most days within a week [83].

Considering the aim of the study, PA measurements were conducted in two groups:

- GrS (n=25)-children and adolescents who participated in their daily PA at school according to their educational program and own lifestyle
- GrR (n=28)-children and adolescents who participated in their daily PA during a rehabilitation summer camp.

The first group of subjects (GrS) were asked to wear an accelerometer for 7 consecutive days, starting on the day immediately after they had received monitors at school. The second group (GrR) was monitored during the second week of a summer camp for children and adolescents with diabetes.

4. Biochemical assessments

Blood samples were collected in the morning using venipuncture after overnight fast. To analyze the children and adolescents' glycemia, the measurements of glucose concentrations, and doses of insulin were repeated 6-8 times per day. The analyses of all individual daily insulin doses were compared to differences in glucose concentrations (Medtronic MiniMed Paradigm 715). Glycated hemoglobin (HbA1c) concentrations were checked (Ames DCA-2000™ Immunoassay Analyzer-normal range: 4.2-6.5%) before and at about two weeks after the end of the study.

For each subject the mean insulin dose and the average blood glucose concentrations were monitored in the morning, afternoon, and evening. Moreover, all incidents of hypo-and hyperglycemia were monitored and recorded and so was the time of their occurrence.

Food intake was recorded and compared to dietary recommendations for all study subjects [32, 84].

Variables	GrS (n=25)	GrR (n=28)
Age [yr]	11.5 (3.4)	12.2 (1.5)
Body height [m]	1.67 (0.1)	1.55 (0.1)
Body mass [kg]	56.0 (9.6)	45.0 (1.0)
BMI [kg/m^2]	19.8 (1.8)	18.9 (2.3)
BMI Centiles[centiles]	51.1 (22.1)	54.5 (23.2)
HgA1c [%]	7.16 (0.38)	7.02 (0.3)

Table 1. Anthropometric and physiologic features of the study population (mean, SD)

http://dx.doi.org/10.5772/57590

5. Statistical analysis

All results are presented as means ± standard deviation. The data were analyzed by two-way ANOVA followed by the Student-Newman-Keuls test when appropriate. Significant differences in glucose concentrations and insulin doses and physical efficiency variables in relation to references ranges were determined using the Bonfferoni post-hock test. Pearson correlation coefficients were analyzed to determine the inter-variable relationships. All analyses were performed using the Statistica v. 9 statistical software package (StatSoft, Tulsa, OK, USA). Statistical significance was set at $p < 0.05$.

6. Results

We studied the effects of energy intake and physical activity on glycaemic control in children and adolescents suffering from diabetes type 1. The variables associated with glucose homeostasis (e.g. daily insulin doses, energy intake, and glycated hemoglobin (HbA1c) were compared during daily activities and in response to exercise/sports participation in a sample of children and adolescents with T1DM.

The assessment of nutritional status of all children and adolescents who participated in the study showed normal body mass and normal BMI percentile values (57.5 ± 20.5 and 52.7 ± 24.9, respectively). Before the study all children had similar levels of hemoglobin A_{1c} (HbA $_{1c}$). Anthropometric features of the two study groups (GrS vs. GrR) were similar for all subjects (Table 1.) Children from the GrS accumulated an average of 8904 ± 981 steps/day while the average activity-induced energy expenditure was 248 ± 40 kcal/day and the relative energy expenditure was 6.06 ± 0.86 kcal/kg/day. The mean number of steps per day during daily PA at school (GrS) was low compared to recommended values (Fig.1).

Analysis of variance revealed a significant effect of physical activity programme during diabetes camp on daily steps ($F=44.0$; $p<0.001$) and daily energy expenditure ($F=21.0$; $p<0.001$). The two-week adherence to a structured exercise programme increased children and adolescents physical activity. Diabetic children who participated in the camp (GrR) accumulated an average of 14378 ± 1699 steps/day, corresponding to 466 ± 48 kcal/day; the relative energy expenditure was 10.4 ± 0.85 kcal/kg/day. A comparison of the study subjects who took part in their daily PA at school according to their educational program (GrS) and participants of the camp for diabetics (GrR) revealed significant differences regarding steps per day ($p<0.001$) and daily energy expenditure ($p<0.01$) between these groups (Table 2).

T1DM children participated in the camp exhibited a higher tolerance of physical exercise on each day of the investigations (Fig. 1). The average daily dose of insulin (Ins/kg) was similar for all subjects, and no significant differences were observed in GrS compared to GrR. No differences were observed in mean daily serum glucose levels between GrS vs GrR groups ($p>0.05$) (Table 2). However, based on the measurements of blood glucose concentrations during the day, several incidents of hypo-and hyperglycemia were observed. Two-way ANOVA revealed a significant effect of physical activity levels on hyperglycemic but not hypoglycemic incidents (GrS vs GrR; $F=1014.7$ $p<0.001$). GrR exhibited a trend to higher number of hypoglycemic events between 10.00 to 12.00 hours compared to GrS (Fig. 2).The number of hyperglycemic events differed depending on the day of the study ($F=442.0$, $p<0.001$). Higher risk of hyperglycemia was noted in children with T1DM who participated in the sports camp. A significant increase in hyperglycemic incidents was diagnosed between 12.00 to 20.00 hours (Fig.3). This trend coincided with the distribution of physical activities carried out during the camp. In the morning we used low-intensity exercise of longer duration while the intensity of afternoon exercises was higher. This might suggest that intense exercise increased the rate of hyperglycemic episodes. A large number of episodes of hyperglycemia directly related to the high intensity exercise may suggest higher glucose levels as a defense mechanism against hypoglycemia.

The analysis of variance indicated a significant effect of the week day on the insulin dose ($F=2.2$; $p<0.05$) with significantly higher doses on Sunday compared to Saturday ($p<0.05$). The average daily glucose concentrations were similar in both groups with a tendency to higher differences in insulin doses in GrR compared to GrS. Sunday results showed an individualized decrease of daily steps, significant increase of insulin doses, and a tendency to hyperglycemia in all investigated diabetics.

Analysis of variance revealed a significant effect of daily energy expenditure during school and rehabilitation programme activities on glycated hemoglobin (HbA1c) concentrations ($F=5.3$; $p<0.05$). A tendency to increased HbA1c levels was observed in GrS after the two weeks of study while GrR subjects had slightly lower levels after the summer camp (Fig. 4).

Participation in a particular study group had a significant effect on fat consumption ($F=15.1$; $p<0.001$) and protein content of the diet ($F=6.9$; $p<0.01$). Children with T1DM from GrR group showed higher fat intakes ($p<0.05$) and lower protein intakes compared to GrS group ($p<0.05$) (Table 3). Protein consumption was higher compared to standard dietary guidelines for children in both GrS and GrR groups (4.7 % vs 2.6% above, respectively). The average values of fat consumption exceeded standard recommendations for children being higher in GrR compared to GrS (9% vs 3.5% above). Carbohydrates consumption was lower than recommended in all investigated diabetics (12% for GrS and 15.3% for GrR below the normal ingestion). Significant correlation was observed between total energy intake and insulin dose ($r=0.57$; $p<0.01$). Lower physical activity was associated with an individualized increase of daily insulin doses in all investigated subjects.

Variables	GrS (n=25)	GrR (n=28)
Energy expenditure [kcal/kg/day]	6.06 (0.86)	10.4 (0.85)**
Average number of steps [steps/day]	8904 (981)	14378 (1699)***
Dose of insulin [u/kg/day]	0.39 (0.03)	0.41 (0.03)
Glucose concentration [mg/dl]	125.1 (8.6)	129.8 (4.5)

**p<0.01; ***p<0.001 significant differences between GrS and GrR.

Table 2. Mean energy expenditure, average number of steps, mean daily dose of insulin, and glucose concentrations on successive week days in the GrS and GrR.

http://dx.doi.org/10.5772/57590

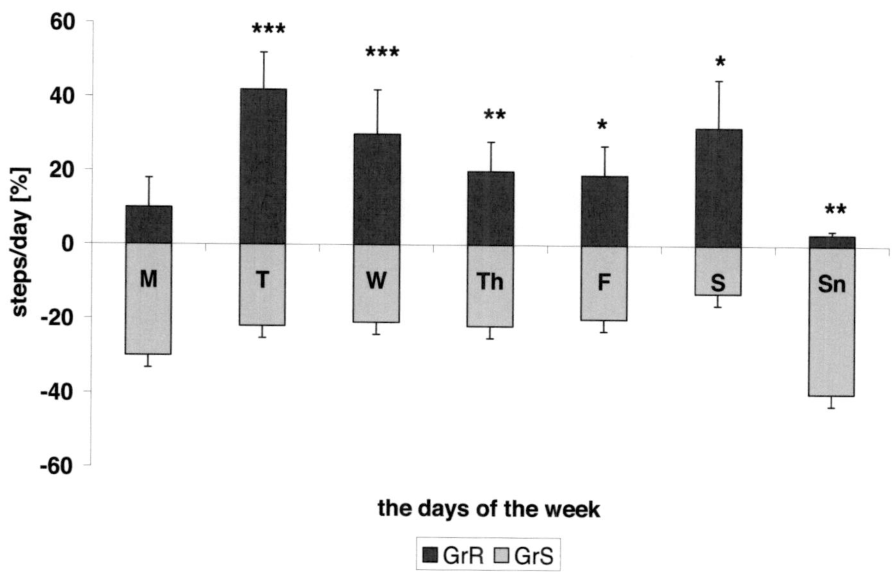

*p<0.05; **p<0.01; ***p<0.001 significant differences between GrS and GrR.

Figure 1. The number of steps compared to the standards in GrS and GrR. (values presented as percentages differences)

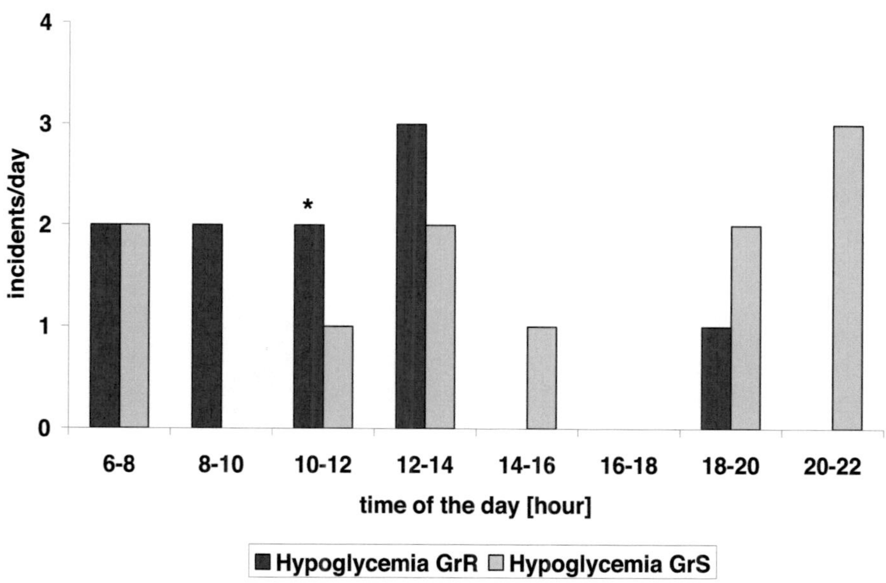

*p<0.05 significant differences between GrS and GrR.

Figure 2. The number of hypoglycemic events at particular time of the day.

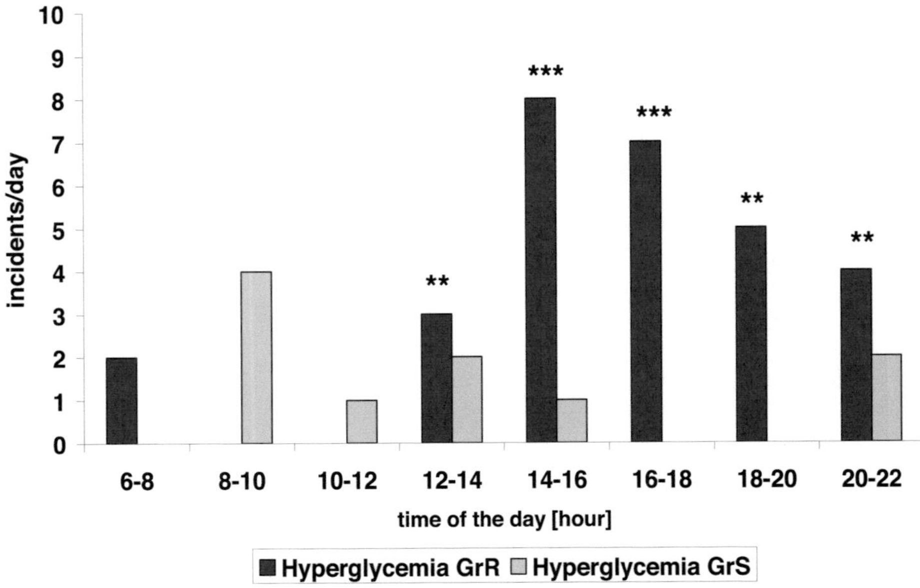

Figure 3. The number of hyperglycemic events at particular time of the day. $^{**}p<0.01$; $^{***}p<0.001$ significant differences between GrS and GrR.

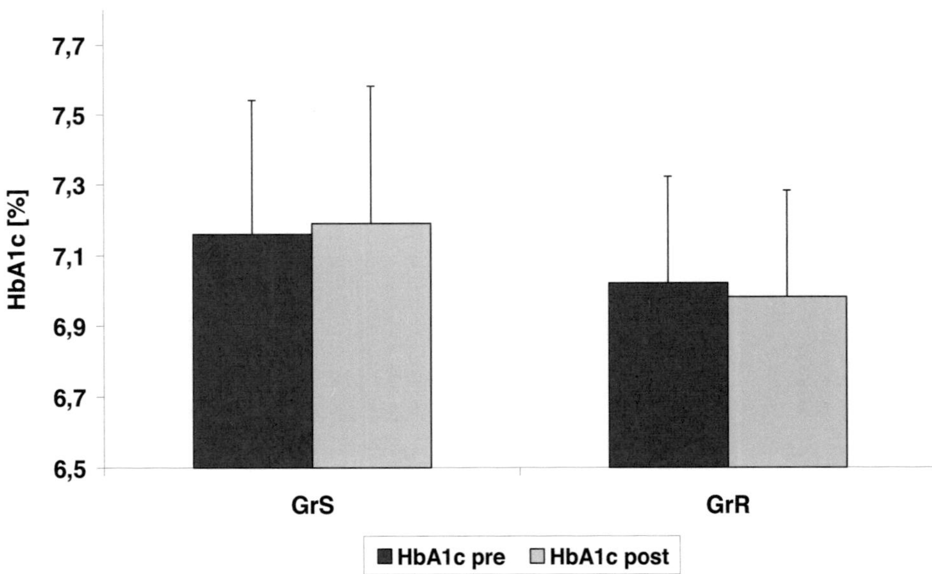

Figure 4. Glycated hemoglobin concentrations (HbA1c%) in GrS and GrR before and after two weeks of study.

http://dx.doi.org/10.5772/57590

Variables	GrS (n=25)	GrR (n=28)
Energy supply with diet [kcal/kg/day]	38.8 (15.6)	35.6 (10.8)
Fat intake [g/kg/day]	1.4 (0.8)	1.7 (0.7)*
Carbohydrate intake [g/kg/day]	3.5 (1.8)	3.2 (1.2)
Protein intake [g/kg/day]	2.1 (1.5)	1.9 (0.8)*

*p<0.05 significant differences between GrS and GrR.

Table 3. Mean energy supply with diet, mean daily fat, carbohydrate, and protein intake on successive days of the week in the GrS and GrR.

7. Discussion

Children and adolescents engage in different types of exercise, most frequently in unplanned and spontaneous physical activities, which can, of course, be associated with immediate and long-term health benefits [36, 62, 85-86]. Children with T1DM gain similar health benefits from physical exercise as their healthy peers; however, due to several consequences of the disease, some specific characteristics of their adaptation to exercise should be considered. Diabetic children and adolescents differ from the healthy pediatric population in their physiological responses to exercise. They are characterized by impaired utilization of exogenous glucose as an energy source during exercise despite hyperinsulinemia and higher rates of perceived exertion, which persist after glucose ingestion [60, 87]. In patients with diabetes, exercise may increases insulin sensitivity and insulin absorption from the site of administration. Plasma glucose levels decrease during and after low-and moderate intensity exercise in response to enhanced glucose utilization in skeletal muscle [88]. In contrast, high-intensity exercise protocols may increase the risk of hyperglycemic episodes [51, 57, 62, 89].

In the present study we analyzed the level of physical activity of children and adolescents with type 1 diabetes and the effect of exercise intensity to compensate blood glucose level depending on the insulin treatment and the diet. Furthermore the aim of the study was to determine the energy expenditure associated with the programmed physical activity which is effective for maintaining normoglycemia in children with type 1 diabetes.

The major findings of our study are that: 1) physical activity in children with type 1 diabetes was lower than the standards for the population of healthy children and recommendations for health training, 2) programmed physical activity significantly increased daily energy expenditure; however, may also increase the risk of hyperglycemia, 3) greater physical activity seemed to provide more effective control of glucose homeostasis as demonstrated by reductions in HbA_{1c}. Our results also show that children with T1DM do not meet the standards of consumption of basic nutrients; higher fat and protein intake with lower carbohydrate values might induce glucose imbalance.

The American Diabetes Association recommends that young patients with diabetes should be given the opportunity to benefit from participating in every type of physical activity, including both recreational and competitive exercises. The understanding of the mechanism of glycemic changes in exercising muscles, modulation of both insulin dose and injection site and appropriate dietary supplementation in T1DM patients prevent the occurrence of adverse events during physical activity [90]. Thus, a thorough understanding of the interactions between exogenous insulin and insulin secretagogues, diet and various forms and intensities of exercise seems to be of great importance to achieve tight metabolic control in diabetic patients. The dose and type of insulin administration (multiple injections/continuous subcutaneous insulin infusion), the site of injection and the timing of insulin dose and food intake before exercise may influence the metabolic and hormonal responses to physical activity among T1DM patients [32, 60, 91].

Plasma glucose concentration is a function of glucose supply, transport rate in the circulation, and metabolism [92-93]. The glucoregulatory hormones, of which insulin is the most important, are designed to maintain circulating glucose concentrations in the physiological range. Initially, insulin stimulates the cells of insulin-sensitive tissues, primarily skeletal muscle, to increase their glucose uptake [6, 43]. Secondly, insulin acts on the liver to inhibit glucose production [42]. The insulin dependent mechanism of glucose transport may be exacerbated by the skeletal muscle contractions. Insulin enhances translocation of specific transporter proteins (GLUT-4) which carry glucose into muscle and adipose cells. In patients with type 1 diabetes mellitus, the insulin-independent mechanism is the most important. Translocation of glucose transporter proteins to cell membrane is initiated by muscle contractions when calcium is released. Recent investigations also indicate that autocrine/paracrine mechanisms observed during exercise (e.g., nitric oxide, adenosine, bradykinin, insulin-like growth hormone-1 may exert alternative or parallel actions [2, 94-96].

It is well established that hypoglycemia is the most common response to exercise; however, in a diabetic patient blood glucose concentrations may also increase or remain unchanged. It is also possible that, even in well-controlled patients, exercise-induced increases in glucose utilization may lead to hypoglycemia [88] both during exercise and up to 31 hours of recovery [90, 97]. Conversely, excessive snacking before exercise, exercise protocols characterized by high intensity and sympathetic nervous systems activation may influence the metabolic response to exercise and increase the risk for hyperglycemia [36, 98]. Several factors may contribute to these adverse reactions during and after exercise [42]. In patients requiring exogenous insulin therapy, insulin levels are predominantly associated with medication; consequently, these levels do not decrease in response to exercise. At the normal exercise-induced decrease in the portal insulin level, hepatic glucose production remains suppressed and cannot increase proportionally to the muscle glucose utilization. As a result, blood glucose declines to hypoglycemic levels [36]. As mentioned above, plasma insulin concentration does not decrease during exercise in T1DM compared to healthy subjects. Quite the opposite-it may even rise, first due to the higher absorption, secondly due to the increased insulin sensitivity, and, finally, in the case when insulin injection is given shortly before exercise. Consequently, the ability to mobilize fat and carbohydrate fuels for exercise may be compromised [3] which facilitates the onset of hypoglycaemia during moderate-intensity exercise [92, 97]. As it was suggested, low-to-moderate intensity exercise was generally recommended for patients with type 1 diabetes since numerous benefits on glucose homeostasis had been observed [91, 95, 99]. However, hypoglycemia can be minimized by appropriately reducing insulin dosage or ingesting additional carbohydrates [60, 90].

Processes regulated by insulin-independent mechanisms are generally preserved when people with diabetes engage in high-intensity exercise. These processes include normal increases in glucose production and disposal during and immediately after the exercise [63, 100-101]. After high-intensity exercise appropriate control of glycaemia is more challenging than in low-intensity exercise due to the role of insulin in modulating the postexercise decline in glucose disposal. Low circulating levels of insulin can prolong hyperglycemia during the recovery after high-intensity exercise, partially counteracting the beneficial effects of exercise on glucose control. If a patient recognizes that a given exercise leads to postexercise hyperglycemia, insulin should be administered shortly after the completion of high-intensity exercise. However, there is evidence that high-intensity exercise, used in combination with low-or moderate-intensity exercise, may maintain blood glucose levels within the normal physiological range and thus minimize the risk of hypoglycemia [62-63].

In the present study, we investigated weekly engagement of children and adolescents with type 1 diabetes in physical activity using an accelerometer. Data regarding their physical activity were obtained through the calculation of mean energy expenditure and compared to reference ranges for children and adolescents. The participants were asked to monitor their physical activity for 7 days during school classes (5 days) and weekend days (2 days). We observed that children and adolescents with T1DM did not adhere to recommended levels of physical activity. Sedentary time was higher on Sunday in all participants and higher in the older group. The proportion of diabetics who did not meet the physical activity recommendations in the present study is consistent with the results of previous studies. Sporting habits in children and adolescents with diabetes were analyzed by Vanelli et al. [102] and Admon et al. [91]. Weekly levels of moderate/vigorous physical activity and sports participation were investigated using a questionnaire. The results showed that children with T1DM appeared to spend less time engaged in physical activity than their non-diabetic peers. Regular physical activity was associated with better metabolic control and lipid profile [103-105]. The association between physical activities, sedentary behavior, and metabolic control in adolescents with T1DM was also observed by Åman et al. [11], who reported that PA was associated with positive health perception but not with glycaemic control, frequency of hypoglycemia or other beneficial effects. In youth with T1DM, prolonged moderate aerobic exercise results in a consistent reduction in plasma glucose and frequent occurrence of hypoglycemia when pre-exercise glucose concentrations are < 120 mg/dl. It also seems that treatment with 15 g of oral glucose is insufficient to reliably treat hypoglycemia during exercise in children and adolescents [88].

Our results showed significantly higher frequency of hyperglycemic events in GrR compared to GrS, with similar amount of hypoglycemic events. It is worth pointing out that GrR exhibited lower glucose levels in the morning whereas hyperglycemia usually appeared in the afternoons and evenings. This coincided with the distribution of physical activities during the camp. In the morning children performed low-intensity exercise of longer duration while the intensity of afternoon exercise was higher.

Our investigations revealed that, compared to dietary standards for children, our study participants showed an excessive intake of proteins and fats and very low carbohydrate intake. Children with T1DM do not meet the standards of basic nutrients consumption [106]. The energy intake from proteins, fat and of carbohydrates compared to dietary standards for children showed an excessive intake of proteins and fats and very low carbohydrate intake. The analysis of variance showed a significant effect of age on the level of fat consumption and positive correlation between the value of energy intake and insulin dose.

Increased intake of fat and protein and lower carbohydrate values can cause problems with insulin administration in response to diet and/or physical activity.

It should be mentioned, that proper nutrition is important in the prevention and treatment of chronic complications of diabetes [107-110]. According to clinical guidelines [71] 40-50% of energy should provide carbohydrate diet, especially a low glycemic index (<50 IG), the fats should provide 30-35% of the energy value of the diet; and protein should be 15-20 %. The ratio of animal protein to vegetable protein should be at least 50/50%. For important recommendations should supplement meals with fluids, vitamins, minerals and fiber [32]. Despite the important role of a balanced diet in the treatment of T1DM, standard recommendations that could help clinicians manage glycemia during exercise are still lacking [111]. The type, duration, and timing of exercise as well as its temporal relation to meals and premeal insulin doses may affect glucose homeostasis during and after exercise. Moreover, regulation of blood glucose associated with physical exercise and anabolic hormonal secretion could be important for long-term glycemic control [112-113]. In the above mentioned studies glycated hemoglobin (HbA1c) could be a better index of long-term glucose homeostasis than measuring fasting and/ or post-challenge glucose [69-70, 73].

The results of the previous study suggested improvement in long-term glycemic control in T1DM youth after a programme of physical activity [10, 105] associated with an increase in aerobic capacity or fitness. Austin et al. [103] also observed a negative correlation between aerobic physical effort and HgA1c levels and daily insulin doses in diabetic patients.

Consistent with these findings, our data also indicated a tendency to HbA1c levels increase in children with lower physical activity (GrS) compared to summer camp participants (GrR).

Our results also demonstrate that participation in an organized rehabilitation programme increased the daily energy expenditure and was associated with tendency to lowering indices of long term glycaemic control (HbA1c%) compared to pretraining levels. This study has limitations that need to be considered before interpreting the findings. The rehabilitation programme might have been too short to significantly improve glycemic control which could be documented by decrease HbA1c level. Also, since the baseline HbA1C levels were slightly over the reference range, ie., below 7.2%, the effects of physical activity in GrR were not so spectacular.

There is evidence that high-intensity exercise along with low-or moderate-intensity exercise might be recommended to diabetic patients. The most important exercise-related benefits in patients with T1DM include reduced serum glucose levels, improved insulin sensitivity and lipid profile, reduced daily dosage of insulin, improved cardiovascular function, reduced body weight and fat accumulation, increase in physical efficiency, and quality of life improvement. Thus, parents, physical education teachers and physical therapists should motivate type 1 diabetic children to engage in physical activity, and supervise them during exercise in order to create a proper approach to physical exercise and reduce the risk for exercise-related complications [110-114].

It should be emphasized that, general exercise recommendations for children and adolescents with T1DM are that they should exercise systematically, for about 30 to 60 minutes, four to five times a week at a low to moderate intensity [115]. In this way they utilize glucose slowly and the effects of preferential fat oxidation improve. Apart from aerobic exercises, diabetics should perform intermittent high-intensity exercise to minimize the occurrence of hypoglycemic events. High-intensity physical exercise causes severe lactic acidosis and increases adrenergic system activation as compared to low-intensity exercise. Consequently, endurance sports activities performed under aerobic threshold are recommended for T1DM patients [98]. On the other hand, a combination of moderate-and high-intensity exercise, a pattern of physical activity referred to as intermittent high-intensity exercise, may also be recommended for youth with T1DM [61, 63, 116]. It is worth to point out that, individual insulin administration scheme (insulin injections and pump) and blood glucose monitoring are of great importance [91]. The authors mentioned that the pump should be removed or turned off during unplanned prolonged exercise to reduce the risk of hypoglycemia.

8. Conclusions

Regular physical activity is an essential element in blood glucose regulation for children and adolescents with type 1 diabetes mellitus. The obtained results indicate that children with type 1 diabetes are not meeting recommended physical activity and dietary guidelines, and especially regarding fat intake. Regular physical activity with high energy expenditure may effectively control glucose homeostasis as documented by HbA_{1c} reduction. However, incorrect dietary behaviors and/or exercise load in T1DM patients may increase the risk of hypo-or hyperglycemia and long-term metabolic complications.

Author details

Aleksandra Żebrowska[1*], Marcin Sikora[1], Przemysława Jarosz-Chobot[2], Barbara Głuchowska[1] and Michał Plewa[3]

*Address all correspondence to: a.zebrowska@awf.katowice.pl

1 Department of Physiological and Medical Sciences, Academy of Physical Education, Katowice, Poland

2 Department of Pediatrics, Endocrinology and Diabetes, Medical University of Silesia, Katowice, Poland

3 Department of Physiotherapy in Internal Diseases, Academy of Physical Education, Katowice, Poland

References

[1] American Diabetes Association. Diagnosis and classification of diabetes mellitus. Diabetes Care 2011; 34(1): 62-9.

[2] Colberg S. Physical activity, insulin action, and diabetes prevention and control. Current Diabetes Review 2007; 3:176-84.

[3] Turcotte LP, Fisher JS. Skeletal muscle insulin resistance: roles of fatty acid metabolism and exercise. Physical Therapy 2008;88:1279-96.

[4] Di Marzio D, Mohn A, Mokini Z, Giannini C, Chiarelli F. Macroangiopathy in adults and children with diabetes: from molecular mechanisms to vascular damage (part 1). Hormone and Metabolic Research 2006;38(11):691-705.

[5] Herbst A, Kordonouri O, Schwab KO, Schmidt F, Holl R. Impact of physical activity on cardiovascular risk factors in children with type 1 diabetes. Diabetes Care 2007;30: 2098-2100.

[6] Holten MK, Zacho M, Gaster M, Juel C, Wojtaszewski JFP, Dela F. Strength training increases insulin-mediated glucose uptake, GLUT-4 content, and insulin signaling in skeletal muscle in patients with type 2 diabetes. Diabetes 2004;53: 294-305.

[7] Giannini C, Giorgis T, Mohn A, Chiarelli F. Role of physical exercise in children and adolescents with diabetes mellitus. Journal of Pediatric Endocrinology & Metabolism 2007; 20: 173-84.

[8] Maiorana A, O'Driscoll G, Goodman C. Combined aerobic and resistance exercise improves glycemic control and fitness in type 2 diabetes. Diabetes Research and Clinical Practice 2002;56: 115-23.

[9] Riddel MC, Iscoe KE. Physical activity, sport and pediatric diabetes. Pediatric `Diabetes 2006;7: 60-70.

[10] Robertson K, Adolfsson P, Riddell M, Scheiner G, Hanas R. Exercise in children and adolescents with diabetes. ISPAD Clinical practice consensus guidelines 2006-2007. Pediatric Diabetes 2008; 9: 65-77.

[11] Åman J, Skinner T, de Beaufort C, Swift P, Aanstoot H, Cameron F. Associations between physical activity, sedentary behavior, and glycemic control in a large cohort of adolescents with type 1 diabetes: the Hvidoere Study Group on Childhood Diabetes. Pediatric Diabetes 2009; 10(4): 234-239.

[12] Galassetti P, Iwanaga K, Crisostomo M, et al. Inflammatory blood glucose and physiological cytokine, growth factor and counterregulatory responses to exercise in children with type 1 diabetes and healthy controls. Pediatric Diabetes 2006;7: 16-24.

[13] American Diabetes Association. Diagnosis and classification of diabetes mellitus. Diabetes Care 2011;34 (1): 62-9.

[14] Daneman D. Type 1 diabetes. Lancet 2006;367: 847-858.

[15] Jahromi MM, Eisenbarth GS. Cellular and molecular pathogenesis of type 1A diabetes. Cellular and Molecular Life Sciences 2007;64; 865-72.

[16] Craig M, Glastras S. Donaghue K. Definition, epidemiology and classification of diabetes and structure of the diabetes team. Allgrove J, Swift PGF, Greene S. Evidence-Based Pediatric and Adolescent Diabetes, Blackwell Publishing, 2007: 9-25.

[17] American Diabetes Association. Diagnosis and classification of diabetes mellitus Diabetes Care 2006;29(1), 43-8.

[18] Karvonen M, Viik-Kajander M, Moltchanova E, Libman I, LaPorte R, Tuomilehto J. Incidence of child-hood type 1 diabetes. Diabetes Care 2000;23: 1516-26.

[19] Nakayama M, Abiru N, Moriyama H, Babaya N, Liu E, Miao D, Yu L, Wegmann DR, Hutton JC, Elliott JF, et al. Prime role for an insulin epitope in the development of type 1 diabetes in NOD mice. Nature 2005; 435: 220-3.

[20] Pirot P, Cardozo A, Eizirik D. Mediators and mechanisms of pancreatic beta-cell death in type 1 diabetes. Arquivos Brasileiros de Endocrinologia e Metabologia 2008; 52(2): 156-165.

[21] Pietropaolo M, Towns R, Eisenbarth GS. Humoral autoimmunity in type 1 diabetes: prediction, significance, and detection of distinct disease subtypes. Cold Spring Harbor Perspectives in Medicine 2012;2:a012831.

[22] Desphande AD, Harris-Hayes M, Schootman M. Epidemiology of diabetes and diabetes-related complications. Physical Therapy 2008; 88: 1224-64.

[23] Achenbach P, Bonifacio E, Koczwara K, Ziegler A. Natural History of Type 1 Diabetes 2005;54(2): 25-31.

[24] Knip M, Siljander H. Autoimmune mechanisms in type 1 diabetes. Autoimmunity Reviews 2008;7(7): 550-557.

[25] Barrett JC, Clayton DG, Concannon P, Akolkar B, Cooper JD, Erlich HA, Julier C, Morahan G, Nerup J, Nierras C, et al. Genome-wide association study and meta-analysis find that over 40 loci affect risk of type 1 diabetes. Nature Genetics 2009;41: 703-7.

[26] Eisenbarth GS. Update in type 1 diabetes. Journal of Clinical Endocrinology & Metabolism 2007;92: 2403-7.

[27] Bluestone JA, Herold K, Eisenbarth GS. Genetics, pathogenesis and clinical interventions in type 1 diabetes. Nature 2010;464: 1293-1300.

[28] Erlich A, Valdes AM, Noble JA. Prediction of type 1 diabetes. Diabetes 2013; 62: 1020-1.

[29] Bangstad H, Danne T, Deeb L, Jarosz-Chobot P, Urakami T, Hanas R. ISPAD Clinical Practice Consensus Guidelines 2006-2007. Insulin treatment. Pediatric Diabetes 2007; 8(2): 88-102.

[30] Alemzadeh R, Palma-Sisto P, Parton E, Totka J, Kirby M. Beneficial effects of flexible insulin therapy in children and adolescents with type 1 diabetes mellitus. Acta Diabetologica 2003;40(3): 137-142.

[31] Toni S, Reali MF, BarniF, Lenzi L, Festini F. Managing insulin therapy during exercise in Type 1 diabetes mellitus. Acta Biomedica 2006;77(1): 34-40.

[32] American Diabetes Association. Standards of medical care in diabetes-2007. Diabetes Care 2007;30(1): 4-41.

[33] Newton K, Wiltshire E, Elley C. Pedometers and text messaging to increase physical activity. Randomized controlled trial of adolescents with type 1 diabetes. Diabetes Care 2009;32: 813-5.

[34] Ruzic L, Sporis G, Matkovic B. High volume-low intensity exercise camp and glycemic control in diabetic children. Journal of Pediatrics and Child Health 2008;44: 122-8.

[35] Australian Pediatric Endocrine Group: Best Practice Guidelines for the Management of Type 1 Diabetes in Children and Adolescents. Performed by Queensland Health's Diabetes Allied Health Task Group, Sydney, AU; 2002. www.health.qld.gov.au/publications/best_practice/

[36] Gulve EA. Exercise and glycemic control in diabetes: benefits, challenges, and adjustments to pharmacotherapy. Physical Therapy 2008;88: 1297-321.

[37] Wilmore JH, Costill DL. Obesity, diabetes, and physical activity. In: Physiology of sport and exercise. J.K.Wilmore, DL. Costill (Ed.), Human Kinetics. 2004: 664-88.

[38] Riddell MC, Perkins BA. Type 1 diabetes and exercise-Part I: Applications of exercise physiology to patient management during vigorous activity. Canadian Journal of Diabetes 2006;30: 63-71.

[39] Wojtaszewski JFP, Richter EA. Glucose utilization during exercise: influence of endurance training. Acta Physiologica Scandinavica 1998;162: 351-8.

[40] Katz A., Sahlin K. Role of oxygen in regulation of glycolysis and lactate production in human skeletal muscle. Exerc. And Sport Sci. Rev. 1990; 18: 1-28.

[41] Brooks G.A., Mercier J. Balance of carbohydrate and lipid utilization during exercise: The "crossover" concept. Journal of Applied Physiology 1994;76: 2253-61.

[42] Camacho R, Galassetti P, Davis S, Wasserman D. Glucoregulation during and after exercise in healthy and insulin dependent diabetes. Exercise and Sport Sciences Reviews 2005;33: 17-23.

[43] Richter EA, Nielsen JN, Jorgensen SB, Frosig C, Wojtaszewski JFP. Signaling to glucose transport in skeletal muscle during exercise. Acta Physiologica Scandinavica 2003;178: 329-35.

[44] Muniyappa R, Lee S, Chen H, Quon MJ. Current approaches for assessing insulin sensitivity and resistance in vivo: advantage, limitations, and appropriate usage. American Journal of Physiology Endocrinology and Metabolism 2008;294: 15-26.

[45] Scheepers A, Joost H, Schürmann A. The glucose transporter families SGLT and GLUT: molecular basis of normal and aberrant function. Silver Spring Journal of Parenteral and Enteral Nutrition 2004;28: 364-372.

[46] Stuart C, Wen G, Williamson M. Altered GLUT1 and GLUT3 gene expression and subcellular redistribution of GLUT4: protein in muscle from patients with acanthosis nigricans and severe insulin resistance. Metabolism 2001;50: 771-777.

[47] Staron RS, Johnson P. Myosin polymorphism and differential expression in adult human skeletal muscle. Comparative Biochemistry and Physiology. Part B 1993; 106: 463-75.

[48] Romijn JA, Coyle EF, Sidossis LS, Gastaldelli A, Horowitz JF, Endert E, Wolf RR. Regulation of endogenous fat and carbohydrate metabolism in relation to exercise intensity and duration. American Journal of Physiology 1993;265: 380-91.

[49] Turcotte LP. Skeletal muscle lipid metabolism during exercise. In: Exercise Metabolism. M. Hargreaves, L.Spriet (Ed.), Human Kinetics Publishers 2006, 105-136.

[50] Cerny FJ, Burton HW. Metabolism In: Exercise Physiology for Health care Professionals. Human Kinetics, Champaign, IL, 2001; 39-57.

[51] Kjaer M, Hollenbeck CB, Frey-Hewit B. Glucoregulation and hormonal responses to maximal exercise in non-insulin-dependent diabetes. Journal of Applied Physiology 1990;68: 2067-74.

[52] Górski J. Muscle triglyceride metabolism during exercise. Acta Physiologica Polonica 1977; 28: 505-10.

[53] Greenhaff PL, Nevill ME, Soderlund K, Bodin K, Boobis LH, Williams C, Hultman E. The metabolic responses of human type I and II muscle fibers during maximal treadmill sprinting. The Journal of Physiology 1994;478: 149-55.

[54] McArdle WD, Katch FI, Katch VL. Energy balance, exercise, and weight control. Sports and Exercise Nutrition, 3rd (Ed.), Lippincott Williams & Wilkins, Philadelphia 2009, 451-91.

[55] Bruss M, Arias E, Lienhard G, Cartee G. Increased phosphorylation of Akt substrate of 160 kDa (AS160) in rat skeletal muscle in response to insulin or contractile activity. Diabetes 2005;54: 41-50.

[56] Zinman B, Ruderman N, Campaigne B, Devlin J, Schneider S. Physical activity/exercise and diabetes. Diabetes Care 2004;27(1): 58-62.

[57] Marliss E, Vranic M. Intense exercise has unique effects on both insulin release and its roles in glucoregulation. Diabetes 2002;51(1): 271-283.

[58] Goodpaster B., Brown N. Skeletal muscle lipid and its association with insulin resistance: what is the role for exercise? Exercise and Sport Science Reviews 2005;33: 150-4.

[59] Francescato MP, Geat M, Fusi S. Carbohydrate requirement and insulin concentration during moderate exercise in type 1 diabetic patients. Metabolism 2004;53: 1126-30.

[60] Riddel MC, Bar-Or O, Ayub BV. Glucose ingestion matched with total carbohydrate utilization attenuates hypoglycaemia during exercise in adolescents with IDDM. International Journal of Sport Nutrition and Exercise Metabolism 1999; 9: 24-34.

[61] Guelfi KJ, Jones TW, Fournier PA. New insights into managing the risk of hypoglycaemia associated with intermittent high-intensity exercise in individuals with type 1 diabetes mellitus. Sports Medicine 2007;37: 937-46.

[62] Guelfi KJ, Jones TW, Fournier PA. The decline in blood glucose levels is less with intermittent high-intensity compared with moderate exercise in individuals with type 1 diabetes. Diabetes Care 2005;28: 1289-94.

[63] Guelfi KJ, Ratnam N, Smythe GA. Effect of intermittent high-intensity compared with continuous moderate exercise on glucose production and utilization in individuals with type 1 diabetes. American Journal of Physiology: Endocrinology and Metabolism 2007;292: 865-70.

[64] Nader P, Bradley R, Houts R, McRitchie S, O'Brien M. Moderate-to-Vigorous Physical Activity From Ages 9 to 15 Years JAMA 2008;300(3): 295-305.

[65] Sigal RJ, Purdon C, Fisher SJ. Hyperinsulinemia prevents prolonged hyperglycaemia after intense exercise in insulin-dependant diabetic subjects. Journal of Clinical Endocrinology & Metabolism 1994;79: 1049-57.

[66] Lenhard MJ, Reeves GD. Continuous subcutaneous insulin infusion. A comprehensive review of insulin pump therapy. Archives of Internal Medicine 2001;161: 2293-300.

[67] Marrone S, White Plume J, Kerr P, Pianol A, Vogeltanz-Holm N, Holm J, Larsen MA. The role of free-play physical activity in healthy blood glucose maintenance in children with type 1 diabetes mellitus. Psychology, Health & Medicine 2009; 14(1):48-52.

[68] Lowes L. Managing type 1 diabetes in childhood and adolescence. Nursing Standard 2008;22(44): 50-6.

[69] Soranzo N. Genetic determinants of variability in glycated hemoglobin (HbA1c) in humans: review of recent progress and prospects for use in diabetic care. Current Diabetes Reports 2011; 11: 562-9.

[70] Nathan DM, Singer DE, Hurxthal K, Goodson JD. The clinical information value of the glycosylated hemoglobin assay. The New England Journal of Medicine 1984; 310: 341-6.

[71] Executive summary: standards of medical care in diabetes-2010. Diabetes Care 2010; 33(1): 4-10.

[72] International expert committee report on the role of the A1C assay in the diagnosis of diabetes. (2009) Diabetes Care 32:1327-34.

[73] Singer GE, Coley CM, Samet JH, Nathan DM. Tests of glycemia in diabetes mellitus. Their use in establishing a diagnosis and in treatment. Annals of Internal Medicine 1989;110: 125-37.

[74] DIAMOND Project Group. Incidence and trends of childhood type 1 diabetes worldwide 1990-1999, Diabetic Medicine 2006;23(8): 857-66.

[75] Miculis CP., Mascarenhas LP., Boguszewski MC, deCampos W. Physical activity in children with type 1 diabetes. Journal of Pediatric, 2010; 86: 271-8.

[76] Mitchell T, Abraham G, Schiffrin A. Hyperglycemia after intense exercise in IDDM subjects during continuous subcutaneous insulin infusion. Diabetes Care 1988; 11(4): 311-7.

[77] O'Neill J, Liese A, Dabelea D. Physical activity and self-concept: the SEARCH for diabetes in youth case control study. Pediatric Exercise Science 2012;24(4): 577-88.

[78] Nagy E. Vicente-Rodriguez G, Manios Y et al. Harmonization process and reliability assessment of anthropometric measurements in a multicenter study in adolescents. International Journal of Obesity (Lond) 2008;32(5):58-65.

[79] Cole TJ, Bellizzi MC, Flegal KM. et al. Establishing a standard definition for child overweight and obesity worldwide: international survey. British Medical Journal 2000; 320 (7244): 1240-3.

[80] Tudor-Locke C, Myers A. Methodological considerations for researchers and practitioners using pedometers to measure physical (ambulatory) activity. Research Quarterly for Exercise & Sport 2001;72: 1-12.

[81] De Greef K, Deforche B, De Bourdeaudhuij I. The effects of a pedometer-based behavioral modification program with telephone support on physical activity and sedentary behavior in type 2 diabetes patients. Patient Education & Counseling 2011;84(2): 275-279.

[82] Physical Activity Guidelines Advisory Committee: Physical Activity Guidelines Advisory Committee Report, 2008. Washington, D.C.: U.S. Department of Health and Human Services 2008.

[83] Tudor-Locke, C., Craig C., Beets M. How many steps/day are enough? For children and adolescents. The International Journal of Behavioral Nutrition and Physical Activity 2011;8(1): 78-84.

[84] Clinical Recommendations for the management of patients with diabetes in 2013. Clinical Diabetology 2013; 2 (A).

[85] Ekblom B, Åstrand PO. Role of physical activity on health in children and adolescents. Acta Pediatrica 2000; 89: 762-74.

[86] Hayes Ch, Kriska A. Role of Physical activity in diabetes management and prevention. Journal of the American Dietetic Association 2008;108(1): 19-23.

[87] Riddell MC, Bar-Or O. American Diabetes Association. Handbook of Exercise in Diabetes: Children and Adolescents. Editors: N. Ruderman, J.T. Devlin, S.H. Schneider., American Diabetes Association 2002;547-66.

[88] Tansey MJ, Tsalikian E, Beck RW, Mauras N, Buckingham BA, Weinzimer SA, Janz KF, Kollman C, Xing D, Ruedy KJ, Steffes MW, Borland TM, Singh RJ, Tamborlane WV. The Diabetes Research in Children Network (DirecNet) Study Group. The effects of aerobic exercise on glucose and counterregulatory hormone concentrations in children with type 1 diabetes. Diabetes Care 2006;29(1): 20-5.

[89] Harmer AR, Chisholm DJ, McKenna MJ, et al. High-intensity training improves plasma glucose and acid-base regulation during intermittent maximal exercise in type 1 diabetes. Diabetes Care 2007; 30: 1269-71.

[90] Rabasa-Lhoret R, Bourque J, Ducros F, Chiasson JL. Guidelines for premeal insulin dose reduction for postprandial exercise of different intensities and durations in type

1 diabetic subjects treated intensively with a basal bolus insulin regimen (Ultra-Lispro). Diabetes Care 2001;24: 625-30.

[91] Admon G, Weinstein Y, Falk B, Weintrob N. Exercise with and without an insulin pump among children and adolescents with type 1 diabetes mellitus. Pediatrics 2005;116: 348-55.

[92] Ertl AC, Davis SN. Evidence for a vicious cycle of exercise and hypoglycaemia in type 1 diabetes Mellitus. Diabetes Metabolism Research and Reviews 2004;20: 124-30.

[93] Bergman RN, Ider YZ, Bowden CR, Cobelli C. Quantitative estimation of insulin sensitivity. American Journal of Endocrinology & Metabolism 1979;236: 667-77.

[94] Bergerot I, Fabien N, Thivolet C. Effects of insulin-like growth factor-1 and insulin on effectors T cells generating autoimmune diabetes. Diabetes Metabolism 1996; 22: 235-9.

[95] Chen W, Salojin KV, Mi Q, Grattan M, Meagher TC, Zucker P, Delovitch TL. Insulin-like growth factor (IGF-)I/IGF-binding protein complex: therapeutic efficacy and mechanism of protection against type 1 diabetes. Endocrinololgy 2004;145: 627-38.

[96] Dunger DB, Cheetham TD. Growth hormone insulin-like growth factor I axis in insulin-dependent diabetes mellitus. Hormonal Research 1996;46: 2-6.

[97] Sandoval DA, Guy DL, Richardson MA, Ertl AC, Davis SN. Effects of low and moderate antecedent exercise on counterregulatory responses to subsequent hypoglycaemia in Type 1 Diabetes. Diabetes 2004;53: 1798-806.

[98] The Diabetes Research in Children Network Study Group. Prevention of hypoglycaemia during exercise in children with type 1 diabetes by suspending basal insulin. Diabetes Care 2006;29: 2204-6.

[99] Plotnikoff RC, Taylor LM, Wilson PM, Courneya KS, Sigal RJ, Birkett N. Factors associated with physical activity in Canadian adult with diabetes. Medicine & Science of Sports & Exercise 2006;38: 1526-34.

[100] Bussau VA, Ferreria LD, Jones TW. The 10-s maximal sprint: a novel approach to counter an exercise mediated fall in glycaemia in individuals with type 1 diabetes. Diabetes Care 2006;29: 601-6.

[101] Grimm JJ, Ybarra J, Bernè C. A new table for prevention of hypoglycaemia during physical activity in type 1 diabetic patients. Diabetes Metabolism 2004;30: 465-70.

[102] Vanelli M, Corchia M, Iovane B, Bernardini A, Mele A, Chiari G. Self-monitoring adherence to physical activity in children and adolescents with type 1 Diabetes 2006;77: 47-50.

[103] Austin A, Warty V, Janosky J, Arslanian S. The relationship of physical fitness to lipid and lipoprotein(a) levels in adolescents with IDDM. Diabetes Care 1993;16: 421-5.

[104] Valerio G, Spaqnuolo MI, Lombardi F, Spadaro R, Siano M, Frazese A. Physical activity and sports participation in children and adolescents with 1 diabetes mellitus. Nutrition Metabolism &Cardiovascular Diseases 2007;17(5): 376-82.

[105] Hawley JA, Lessard SJ. Exercise training-induced improvements in insulin action. Acta Physiologica (Oxf.) 2008:192, 127-35.

[106] Sarnblad S, Ekelund U, Aman J. Physical activity and energy intake in adolescent girls with type 1 diabetes. Diabetes Medicine 2005;22: 893-9.

[107] Schweiger B, Klingensmith G, Snell-Bergeon J. Physical Activity in Adolescent females with Type 1 Diabetes. International Journal of Pediatrics, 2010; 10.1155/2010/328318

[108] D'hooge R, Hellinckx T, Calders P. Influence of combined aerobic and resistance training on metabolic control, cardiovascular fitness and quality of life in adolescents with type 1 diabetes: a randomized controlled trial. Clinical Rehabilitation 2011; 25(4): 349-59.

[109] Franz M, Bantle J, Beebe C, Brunzell J, Chiasson J, Garg A, Holzmeister L, Hoogwerf B, Mayer-Davis E, Mooradian A. Evidence based nutrition principles and recommendations for the treatment and prevention of diabetes and related complications. Diabetes Care 2002;25: 148-9.8

[110] Wareham NJ. Epidemiological studies of physical activity and diabetes risk, and implication for diabetes prevention. Applied Physiology Nutrition & Metabolism 2007; 32: 778-82.

[111] Guelfi KJ, Jones TW, Fournier PA. Intermittent high-intensity exercise does not increase risk of early postexercise hypoglycaemia in individuals with type 1 diabetes. Diabetes Care 2005;28: 416-8.

[112] Tamborlane WV, Sherwin RS, Koivisto V, Hendler R, Genel M, Felig P. Normalization of the growth hormone and catecholamine response to exercise in juvenile-onset diabetic subjects treated with a portable insulin infusion pump. Diabetes 1979;28: 785-8.

[113] Adolfsson P, Nilsson S, Albertsson-Wikland K, Lindblad B. Hormonal response during physical exercise of different intensities in adolescents with type 1 diabetes and healthy controls. Pediatric Diabetes 2012;13(8): 587-96.

[114] Wolfsdorf JI. Children with diabetes benefit from exercise. Archives of Disease of Childhood 2005; 90: 1215-7.

[115] Lumb AN, Gallen IW. Insulin dose adjustment and exercise in type 1 diabetes: what do we tell the patients. British Journal Diabetes & Vascular Diseases. 2009;9: 273-277.

Chapter 4

Role of Magnesium in the Regulation of Hepatic Glucose Homeostasis

Chesinta Voma and Andrea M.P. Romani

Additional information is available at the end of the chapter

http://dx.doi.org/10.5772/57564

1. Introduction

1.1. The liver and glucose metabolism

The liver comprises of hepatocytes, biliary epithelial cells, stellate cells (or Ito cells), Kupffer cells, sinusoid endothelial cells, and pit cells [1,2]. Most of the clinically quantifiable liver functions such as metabolic processes and protein synthesis take place within the hepatocytes, while non-hepatocyte cells are responsible for other functions including inflammatory response (Kupffer cells), collagen deposition (Ito cells), and cell orientation [2-5]. Regulation of blood glucose is one of the main functions exerted by the liver. The organ contains a dynamic storage of glycogen that is rapidly dismissed into the circulation as glucose to maintain glycemia and support brain functions. Hence, hepatocytes are enzymatically specialized to switch rapidly between glycogenolysis and glycogenosynthesis based upon hormonal stimuli and metabolic conditions.

Glucose enters the hepatocytes through the low-affinity transporter GLUT2 (Km=15-20 mM, Table 1). At variance of GLUT1 and GLUT4 glucose transporter that possess a Km=1-5mM and are therefore constitutively active near their maximal rate under euglycemic conditions (i.e. between 60 to 100 mg/dl), GLUT2 is maximally activated following a meal. The high Km of GLUT2 (~15-20mM) correlates well with the high Km glucokinase responsible for the conversion of glucose to glucose 6-phosphate [6].

Glucose 6-phosphate (G6P) can be routed towards glycogenosynthesis, glycolysis, or oxidation by the cytoplasmic glucose 6-phosphate dehydrogenase, *de facto* entering the pentose shunt pathway, an alternative path that generates ribose 5-phosphate utilized in nucleic acid formation (cell cycle) or return as glucose 6-phosphate to be used once again as most convenient for the cell (Fig.1). Glucose 6-phosphate is also transported into the endoplasmic reticulum

Transporter	Affinity for Glucose (Km)	Location
Glut1	1-2 mmol/L	ubiquitous
Glut2	15-20 mmol/L	hepatocytes, β-cells
Glut3	1-2 mmol/L	ubiquitous
Glut4	3.5-8 mmol/L	skeletal muscles, adipocytes

Table 1. Glucose Transporters

to undergo hydrolysis via glucose 6-phophatase, or oxidation via the hexose 6-phosphate dehydrogenase, the reticular variant of the glucose 6-phosphate dehydrogenase [7].

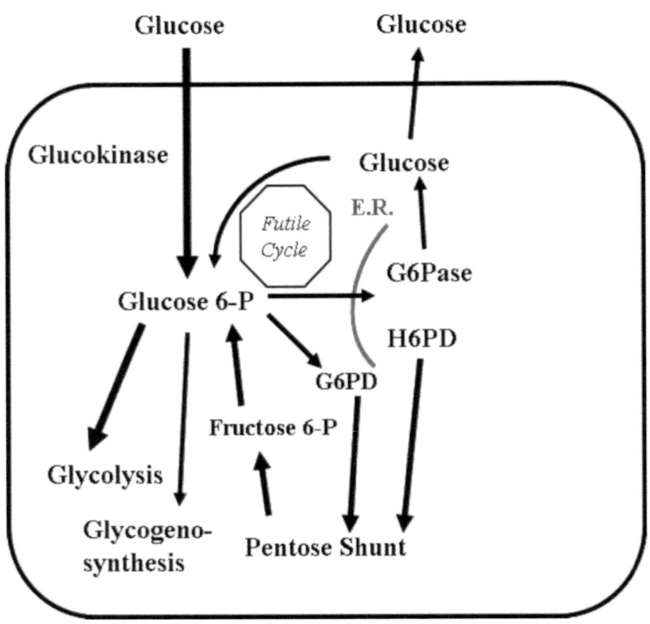

Figure 1. Cartoon depicting the different destinies of glucose 6–phosphate (G6P) within the hepatocyte.

The modality whereby glucose 6-phosphate enters the hepatic E.R. lumen is still debated. The *substrate-transport* theory postulates that G6P enters the ER lumen via a specific transporter (T1) distinct from the glucose 6 phosphatase. In this model, T1 represents the rate-limiting factor for the G6Pase system [8]. The *conformational flexibility substrate-transport* theory proposes that the G6Pase enzyme possesses a hydrophilic region that spans the E.R. membrane and project into the cytoplasm. This region is specific for substrate binding and is distinct from the hydrolytic site. Upon binding to glucose 6-phosphate this cytoplasmic site of the protein undergoes a conformational change and delivers the substrate to the intra-luminal catalytic site. According to this model, the substrate binding site and a hydrolytic site of the G6Pase are two parts of the same protein, and the enzyme is not specific for a particular substrate [9].

Irrespective of the modality of entry, the hydrolysis of glucose 6-phosphate by the hydrolytic site of the glucose 6-phosphatase generates two byproducts, glucose and inorganic phosphate (Pi), which are released into the cytoplasm via two additional, specific transport mechanisms [8-11]. The glucose exported out of the ER is either earmarked for glucose output from the hepatocyte into the bloodstream or is converted anew to glucose 6-phosphate by the glucokinase thereby contributing to the glucose-glucose 6-phosphate *futile* cycle [12]. The inorganic phosphate (Pi) is either exported out of the ER lumen through its specific transporter, or forms a complex with the Ca^{2+}ions that are actively transported into the ER lumen by the SERCA pumps [13]. Far from being static and irreversible, this Ca*Pi complex promotes an enlargement of the reticular Ca^{2+}pool within the hepatocyte, and it can be dynamically reversed to $Ca^{2+}$and Pi, with both moieties being mobilized out of the ER following IP_3–induced Ca^{2+}-release [13]. Thus, this enlargement of the reticular Ca^{2+}pool is an integral part of the hepatic response to hormones such as vasopressin or norepinephrine that tap into the IP_3-related Ca^{2+}-response for metabolic and functional purposes [14].

Further investigation is required to fully elucidate the functional implications of the reticular hexose 6-phosphate dehydrogenase. This enzyme also utilizes the glucose 6-phosphate transported into the E.R., oxidizing it to 6-phosphogluconolactone [7]. Essentially, this enzyme performs the first two steps of the pentose shunt pathway within the E.R. [7.] and is responsible for maintaining a reduced pyridine nucleotide pool ($NADPH/H^+$) within the E.R. to be utilized in various reticular functions including E.R. stress regulation [15]. Presently, it is unknown whether the expression and activity of the hexose 6-phosphate dehydrogenase (H6PD) change as a result of hormonal stimuli, metabolic conditions, or liver pathologies.

The liver plays a critical role in maintaining blood glucose levels within the normal range during the fed-fast cycle. During early fasting, hepatic glycogenolysis and glucose output from the organ maintains glycemia within a suitable range for brain function and metabolism. As the amount of glycogen stored within the liver (i.e. ~10% of the organ weight) is not sufficient to maintain glycemia over an extended period of time or prolonged fasting, gluconeogenesis becomes essential to synthesize glucose from amino acids, lactate and pyruvate dismissed into the circulation by skeletal muscles through glycogenolysis and glycolysis, and from glycerol dismissed by adipose tissue through lipolysis.

The complex metabolic scenario of fed to fast cycling is maintained through the antagonistic roles of insulin on one side, and glucagon, catecholamine and glucocorticoids on the other side. All these hormones modulate liver metabolism through the glucose to glucose 6-phosphate futile cycle [12], with insulin inhibiting the glucose 6-phosphatase activity and expression, and the pro-glycemic hormones increasing them.

During fed and postprandial states, elevation in blood glucose level promptly increases insulin secretion from pancreatic β-cells, which in turn, decreases glucagon release from pancreatic α-cells. The combined effect of these hormonal changes decreases hepatic glucose output and production by suppressing gluconeogenesis and glycogenolysis while increasing glucose storage within skeletal muscles via glycogenosynthesis and adipocytes via lipogenesis. In addition, insulin promotes glucose utilization in peripheral tissues through activation of glycolysis [16].

1.2. Physiological magnesium homeostasis

1.2.1. Cellular magnesium distribution

Our body absorbs minerals through food and drinks consumed daily. However, industrial food processing techniques limit to a varying extent the dietary content and intake of minerals and vitamins, making necessary the utilization of supplements. This is indeed the case of the macro mineral magnesium. Overall, $Mg^{2+}$is the fourth most abundant cation in vertebrates and the second most abundant cation within cells after potassium. In humans, total body magnesium (Mg^{2+}) is found mostly in the bones (60-65% of total content), soft tissues and cells in general [17]. Only 1% of total body magnesium is found in the extracellular fluid, thus making serum magnesium level a poor indicator of total magnesium content and availability in the body. Of the 1% total body Mg^{2+}present in the extracellular fluid, about sixty percent (60%) is free, the reminder (~33%) being bound to proteins, citrate, bicarbonate, ATP[1] and phosphate (≤7%) [18].

Whole body Mg^{2+}homeostasis changes overtime. At an early stage, most Mg^{2+}in the bones can readily exchange with serum, representing an optimal store to compensate for occasional dietary deficiency. As age progresses, however, the proportion of readily exchangeable Mg^{2+}in the bones decreases significantly due to a change in bone crystal size with age [19]. In individuals consuming Mg^{2+}enriched diet, a positive association between bone mineral density and Mg^{2+}content within the erythrocytes has been reported [20].

At the cellular level, $Mg^{2+}$is highly compartmentalized within nucleus, endoplasmic or sarcoplasmic reticulum, mitochondria, and cytoplasm [18], the only notable exception being the erythrocytes, in which $Mg^{2+}$is merely cytoplasmic [21]. In the majority of mammalian cells examined, including the hepatocytes, total cellular Mg^{2+}concentrations range from 15 to 20mM as measured by various techniques including electron X ray microprobe analysis (EXPMA), fluorescent dyes, and scanning fluorescence x-ray microscopy [21]. Total Mg^{2+}concentrations between 15 and 20mM have also been measured within the nucleus, the mitochondria, and the rough endoplasmic reticulum of various cell types by EPXMA [21]. In the cytoplasm, $Mg^{2+}$is present as a complex with ATP (~4-5mM=Mg*ATP) and other phosphonucleotides [22]. Consequently, the free Mg^{2+}concentration ($[Mg^{2+}]_i$) within the cytoplasm and the mitochondrial matrix ranges between 0.5 and 1.2 mM [21,23], i.e. slightly below or at the concentration present in the extracellular environment. These measurements suggest that the majority of mammalian cells are near *zero trans* conditions as far it concerns the cellular distribution of Mg^{2+}.

Despite the large amount of Mg^{2+}present within the majority of mammalian cells, limited information is available about the physiological role of $Mg^{2+}$for specific cell function. In liver cells, Mg^{2+}controls ATP production by the mitochondria and its utilization by various ATPases including the Na^+/K^+-ATPase [21] and the reticular Ca^{2+}-ATPase [21]. As a result, 90% of cytoplasmic ATP is in the form of a complex with Mg^{2+}[24]. Moreover, in hepatocytes $Mg^{2+}$is a cofactor for many enzymes involved in energy metabolism, including glycolysis and Krebs cycle [25]. The list of Mg^{2+}-regulated glycolytic enzymes includes hexokinase, phosphofructokinase, aldolase, phosphoglycerate kinase and pyruvate kinase [26]. The regulation of specific

http://dx.doi.org/10.5772/57564

enzymes or channels by $Mg^{2+}$is not restricted to the cytoplasm occurring also in the cellular organelles in which $Mg^{2+}$is compartmentalized. In liver mitochondria, changes in matrix Mg^{2+}content regulate the activity of succinate and glutamate dehydrogenases but not α-ketoglutarate dehydrogenases [23]. In addition, Mg^{2+}regulates the opening of the inner mitochondrial anion channel (IMAC), the permeability transition pore (PTP), K_{ATP}-channels, and possibly the H^+/K^+exchanger, thus regulating the organelle volume [23]. It is still unresolved as to whether $Mg^{2+}$is required for the adenine nucleotide translocase to operate [23]. At the level of the hepatic rough endoplasmic reticulum (R.E.R.), Mg^{2+}regulates Ca^{2+}uptake via the Ca-ATPase, and its release through the IP_3 receptor [27], as well as the rate of protein synthesis and dismissal into the cytoplasm via the translocon [28]. Experimental evidence suggests that Mg^{2+}inversely regulates the rate of glucose 6-phosphate entry into the E.R. lumen, thus providing higher level of substrate to the glucose 6-phosphatase (G6Pase), and the hexose 6-phosphate dehydrogenase (H6PD) under conditions in which cellular Mg^{2+}levels are reduced [29]. In the nucleus, changes in Mg^{2+}content have been associated with inhibition of specific endonucleases and chromatin folding [21]. Less known is the function of Mg^{2+}within the Golgi lumen. The recent localization of a Mg^{2+}transporter in the Golgi cisternae, however, suggests a possible role of the cation in regulating protein glycosylation [23]. As for endosomal and lysosomal vesicles, nothing is known about the Mg^{2+}concentration within these vesicles and its role in modulating their physiological processes.

Despite its large total concentration within the cell, $Mg^{2+}$is not a static cation. Major Mg^{2+}fluxes have been detected across the cell membrane of the hepatocyte and other mammalian cells. Various hormones and pharmacological agents modulate total and free Mg^{2+}concentrations within the hepatocyte, supporting the hypothesis that many of the metabolic changes elicited by these agents are attained by changing the concentration of Mg^{2+}within the cells and/or within specific cellular compartments, which then results in the up-or down-regulation in the activity of Mg-sensitive enzymes.

1.2.2. Cellular magnesium transport mechanisms

The current understanding of Mg^{2+}transport across the hepatocyte cell membrane indicates that Mg^{2+}exits the liver cell via a Na^+/Mg^{2+}exchanger [30,31], which functionally depends on the physiological concentration of extracellular Na^+[30,32] and the cellular level of cAMP [33], which activates the exchanger through phosphorylation [34]. Under conditions in which limited inward Na^+gradient is present across the cell membrane, or Na^+transport is inhibited by agents like amiloride or imipramine, cellular $Mg^{2+}$is extruded via a Na^+-independent mechanism that utilize different cations or anions in counter-transport for or co-transport with Mg^{2+}, respectively [32].

As for Mg^{2+}entry, hepatocytes appear to utilize predominantly the TRPM7 channel [35]. Protein kinase C (PKC) appears to regulate this channel directly via phosphorylation of its C terminus, or indirectly by removing RACK1-inhibition [36].

Several other Mg^{2+}entry mechanisms have been observed to be present in liver cells [32] but it is still unclear to which extent these mechanism cooperate with TRPM7 in mediating Mg^{2+}entry and in regulating hepatic Mg^{2+}homeostasis.

1.2.3. Regulation of magnesium transport

The specific modality of operation and regulation of the various Mg^{2+}transport mechanisms have been extensively addressed in recent review articles [32,37-39], and we refer to those reviews for further information. For the purpose of this chapter, we will only mention that in liver cells both Mg^{2+}entry and extrusion are under hormonal control. Hormones like catecholamine and glucagon, which increase cAMP level within the hepatocyte, all promote Mg^{2+}extrusion by phosphorylating the Na^+/Mg^{2+}exchanger mentioned above [40]. Activation of α_1-adrenoceptors by catecholamine also induces Mg^{2+}extrusion. Stimulation of this class of adrenergic receptors activates PLCγ, which in turn hydrolyzes phosphatidyl-inositol bisphosphate (PIP2) to diacylglycerol and inositol 1,4,5-trisphosphate (IP_3). The IP_3-induced Ca^{2+}release from the endoplasmic reticulum and the subsequent capacitative Ca^{2+}entry through the hepatocyte plasma membrane promote Mg^{2+}extrusion from the hepatocyte, most likely by displacing $Mg^{2+}$for $Ca^{2+}$from organelle and cytosolic binding sites [41]. This is consistent with the observation that distinct $Na^+$and Ca^{2+}-dependent Mg^{2+}extrusion mechanisms operate in the basolateral and the apical portion of the hepatocyte cell membrane, respectively [34,42]. The differential activation of the Na^+-dependent (β-adrenergic receptors and glucagon receptor) and the Ca^{2+}-dependent Mg^{2+}extrusion mechanism (α_1-adrenergic receptors) points to the ability of the hepatocytes to activate Mg^{2+}extrusion by different modalities and circumvent possible inhibitory mechanisms. It has to be noted, in fact, that insulin pre-treatment abolishes the Mg^{2+}extrusion mediated by cAMP but not that mediated via α_1-adrenoceptor activation [43]. Conversely, hormones or agents that maximize Ca^{2+}release from the ER elicit a time-dependent inhibition of α_1-adrenergic receptor mediated Mg^{2+}extrusion that leaves unaffected the extrusion occurring via β-adrenergic receptors stimulation and cellular cAMP elevation [44]. In this contest, it has to be noted that cytoplasmic free $[Mg^{2+}]$i modulates adenylyl cyclase activation in a variety of cell types including hepatocytes [45]. Under resting conditions, cytoplasmic $[Mg^{2+}]$i is insufficient to activate the adenylyl cyclase maximally. Following β-adrenoceptor or glucagon receptor stimulation the cytoplasmic Mg^{2+}pool increases markedly but transiently via the release of $Mg^{2+}$from other cellular pool (namely mitochondria and endoplasmic reticulum) promoting adenylate cyclase activity and cAMP synthesis [45]. Elevation of cytoplasmic $[Mg^{2+}]$i also inhibits IP_3-induced Ca^{2+}-release [27] most likely via a direct modulatory effect of Mg^{2+}on the IP_3 receptor subunits.

Cellular Mg^{2+}accumulation is also under hormonal regulation. Among the hormones involved in the process there are insulin and vasopressin. These hormones either counteract cAMP production by acting at the level of the β-adrenergic receptor (inhibition) or the cytoplasmic phosphodiesterase that converts cAMP to AMP (stimulation), and/or activate PKC signaling, which acts as cAMP *alter ego*. Due to its ubiquitous presence and abundance, the TRPM7 channel is the mechanism most likely responsible for Mg^{2+}accumulation in the hepatocyte [46]. It is presently unclear whether PKC activates the channel by binding RACK1 and removing this protein from a specific site near the C terminus of the channel through which RACK1 inhibits TRPM7 conductance [36], or whether phosphorylation of the channel C-terminus is also required for full activation [46]. In the case of insulin, a direct modulatory effect on the putative Na^+/Mg^{2+}exchanger has also been observed [47].

Both Mg^{2+}extrusion and Mg^{2+}accumulation are quantitatively and timely limited processes [48,49], implying the movement of $Mg^{2+}$from and to specific cellular compartments. The cytoplasm is but one of the cellular compartments involved in Mg^{2+}transport out of the cell or into the cells [21,22], other compartments being the mitochondria and the endoplasmic reticulum [21]. This notion is supported by the observation that the co-stimulation of hepatic β_2-and α_1-adrenergic receptors by the mix agonist epinephrine results in a Mg^{2+}extrusion that is quantitatively similar to the sum of the Mg^{2+}amounts mobilized by the stimulation of each adrenoceptor class by specific agonists [40]. However, the mechanisms involved in Mg^{2+}transport in-and-out of these compartments have not been fully elucidated. It is known that mitochondria accumulate Mg^{2+}through Mrs2, a Mg^{2+}-specific channel, the absence of which affects complex I expression and activity [50]. Less certain is whether Mg^{2+}extrusion from the mitochondria occurs via the adenine nucleotide translocase [21]. As for the cytoplasm, this compartment acts as a temporary step-in between the extracellular compartment and the cellular organelles both in the extrusion and in the accumulation of Mg^{2+}due to the high concentration of ATP that buffers $Mg^{2+}$with a very high Kd (~75μM) and the presence of other phosphonucleotides and binding proteins [22]. The role of ATP is further supported by the observation that pathological conditions that decrease cellular ATP content through dysmetabolic processes (namely diabetes and alcoholic liver disease) ultimately cause Mg^{2+}loss from the cell [51-53].

2. Insulin signaling in the liver

Insulin signaling is mediated by a complex and highly integrated signaling network that controls several processes including whole body glucose homeostasis. The liver is the first organ 'seen' by insulin following its release from the β-cells into the portal vein, and is responsible for the clearance of 50% of the released insulin at the first pass. Stimulation of the insulin receptor in liver cells is a key event to regulate hepatic glucose homeostasis. In addition, insulin acts indirectly on hepatic glucose homeostasis in that insulin released from β-cells inhibits glucagon release from pancreatic α-cells thus limiting the drive on hepatic gluconeogenesis. The impairment of both these processes observed in insulin resistance is linked to major health problems including type 2-diabetes.

Insulin initiates its signaling cascade by interacting with the insulin receptor on the cell surface. Binding of insulin to the extracellular α-subunits of the insulin receptor results in a conformation change that translates to the intracellular β-subunits of the receptor. The consequent activation of the kinase domain in the β-subunits of the receptor results in the autophosphorylation of specific tyrosine residues in the intracellular β-subunits. The phosphorylated insulin receptor now recruits the insulin receptor susbstrate (IRS), which upon phosphorylation on tyrosine residues acts as a docking unit for numerous cellular proteins including the phosphatidyl inositol 3-kinase (PI3K) [54]. Recruitment of these proteins to the IRS results in their activation. Activation of PI3K results in the phosphorylation of PIP2 to PIP3 and in the subsequent activation of protein kinase B (PKB or Akt), which then phosphorylates Forkhead box protein O1 (FoxO1), preventing its translocation to the nucleus. In its un-phosphorylated state FoxO1 localizes in the nucleus, binds to the insulin response element sequence of gluconeogenesis-related genes, chiefly glucose 6 phosphatase and PEPCK, and increases their transcription rate, indirectly increasing the rate of hepatic glucose production. In its phosphorylated state, FoxO1 is unable to translocate to the nucleus and to activate the gluconeogenesis-related genes. Inhibition of FoxO1 could then improve hepatic metabolism in cases of insulin resistance and metabolic syndrome [55].

2.1. Role of Mg^{2+}on insulin receptor activation and signaling

The human insulin receptor homodimer is heavily glycosylated and contains a total of 19 predicted N-linked glycosylation sites in each monomer. The presence of sialic acid residues on molecules and cells is critical to their biological function and the presence of sialic acid residues on glycoproteins is partly responsible for the binding and transport of molecules, masking of the surface charge, aggregation and shape of cells [56]. Most recently, neuraminidase-1(Neu-1) an enzyme responsible for hydrolyzing sialic acid (neuraminic acid), has been associated with the positive regulation of insulin signaling [57]. Neu-1 is transported to the cell surface and gets involved in the regulation of cell signaling. Insulin binding to its receptor rapidly induces interaction of the glycan chains of the receptor with Neu-1 which hydrolyzes sialic acid residues in the glycan chains of the receptor consequently inducing activation of the insulin receptor. Impaired insulin-induced phosphorylation of Akt, thus identifies Neu1 as a novel component of the signaling pathways of energy metabolism and glucose uptake. Insulin binding to the insulin receptor has been shown to induce the interaction of the receptor with a pool of Neu-1 near the cell surface [57]. Also, insulin signaling is partially impaired in tissues of Neu-1-deficient mice [3], and desialylation of the insulin receptor by Neu1 promote the receptor activation [57]. While $CaCl_2$ has no significant effect on human liver neuraminidase activity, 10mM $MnCl_2$ or $MgCl_2$ shows a mild stimulatory effect (112% and 125% over control activity, respectively) [56].

Additional experimental evidence indicates that $Mg^{2+}$is required for the activated insulin receptor to phosphorylate IRS [54].

3. Magnesium and hepatic glucose metabolism

In liver cells, adrenergic stimulation of α_1-and β-adrenergic receptors, and glucagon receptors elicit a Mg^{2+}extrusion that is associated with activation of glycolysis and glucose output on functional and temporal bases [40]. Although the nature of this association requires further clarification, it is fairly evident that conditions that limit the amplitude of Mg^{2+}extrusion decrease the amount of glucose outputted from liver cells, and vice versa [40]. This association is further supported by several pieces of observation. Overnight starvation, which depletes the liver of its glycogen content, decreases total hepatic Mg^{2+}content by 10-15% [58] rendering liver cells unresponsive to any subsequent adrenergic stimulation [58]. Both type-1 and type-2 diabetes present with a marked decrease in hepatic Mg^{2+}content [59], and treatment with the anti-diabetic drug metformin, which operates predominantly on liver metabolism, increases intra-hepatic Mg^{2+}content [60]. The loss of hepatic Mg^{2+}observed under diabetic conditions depends on the enhanced phosphorylation of the Na^{+}.Mg^{2+}exchanger [61,62], and can be attenuated to a significant extent by the presence of glycogen, amylopectin, or glucose within liver plasma membrane vesicle [62].

The functional association between $Mg^{2+}$and glucose is also observed for Mg^{2+}accumulation. Insulin, one of the hormones involved in Mg^{2+}accumulation, is also responsible for glucose accumulation and conversion to glycogen [58]. Following insulin administration, Mg^{2+}accumulation is directly proportional to the amount of glucose present in the system [63]. Conversely, decreasing Mg^{2+}content in the extracellular system decreased the accumulation of glucose within the cells [40,63]. In part, the limited accumulation of glucose into insulin-stimulated cells in the presence of low extracellular Mg^{2+}concentration can be explained with the reduced activation of the insulin receptor occurring in these cells as $Mg^{2+}$is essential for the proper autophosphorylation of the insulin receptor and the subsequent recruitment of the insulin receptor substrate to the activated receptor [54]. All together, these pieces of evidence and observation support an essential role of Mg^{2+}in glucose regulation and pose for the cation as an important player in the onset and development of insulin resistance and diabetes in human patients.

3.1. Magnesium and enzyme activation in glucose metabolism

The physiological role of magnesium is principally related to enzyme activity. All enzymes utilizing ATP require Mg for substrate formation. Intracellular free magnesium also acts as an allosteric activator of enzyme action including critical enzyme systems such as adenylate cyclase, phosphofructokinase, phospholipase C, and Na^{+}/K^{+}-ATPase [64]. Magnesium is an enzyme substrate (ATPMg, GTPMg) to enzymes such as ATPase (Na^{+}, K^{+}ATPase, Ca^{2+}ATPase), cyclases (adenylate cyclase, guanylate cyclase), and the kinases (hexokinase, protein kinase) [64]. Recently, our laboratory has provided evidence that Mg^{2+}also modulates the amount of glucose 6-phosphate being routed into the endoplasmic reticulum (E.R) to be hydrolyzed to glucose plus Pi by the glucose 6-phosphatase, or to be converted to 6-phosphogluconolactone by the hexose 6-phosphate dehydrogenase, the reticular version of the G6PD. Moreover, our laboratory has provided significant evidence that both glucose and Mg^{2+}homeostasis are altered under pathological conditions such as diabetes [61] and alcoholic liver disease [65].

Many of the enzymes of glycolytic pathway that utilizes glucose have a requirement for Mg^{2+} [26] and utilize $MgATP^{2-}$as a cofactor [66]. The Km values for Mg^{2+}in the glycolytic enzymes of the human erythrocyte are between 1 and 2.3 mM for hexokinase, 0.025 mM for phosphofructokinase (PFK), 0.3 mM for phosphoglycerate kinase (PGK), and 1 mM for pyruvate kinase [26]. Magnesium ions (Mg^{2+}) and $MgATP^{2-}$regulate the most important glycolytic enzymes, namely hexokinase, phosphofructokinase, aldolase, phosphoglycerate kinase, and pyruvate kinase [66]. Glucokinase (Hexokinase IV or D), an enzyme expressed predominantly in liver and pancreatic β-cells of vertebrates, shows marked deviations from Michaelis-Menten kinetics when the glucose concentration is varied at a constant $MgATP^{2-}$concentration, but shows no deviations from Michaelis-Menten kinetics with respect to $MgATP^{2-}$[26,67]. Compared to the other hexokinase isoenzymes, this isoform has a low affinity for glucose (Table

1). Maximum binding of glucokinase and its regulatory protein to the hepatocyte matrix occurs at low [glucose] (<5mM) in a Mg^{2+}-dependent manner (Table 2, [68]). The regulatory protein binds to the hepatocyte matrix with ionic characteristics similar to those of glucokinase but, unlike glucokinase, it does not translocate from the binding site. Since the binding of glucokinase to its regulatory protein is associated with a decrease in the affinity of the enzyme for glucose, the bound enzyme in the presence of Mg^{2+}represents an inactive state and the translocated enzyme a more active state [69].

Substrates	Dissociation Constants (K_d)
0 mM Glucose	0.14 ± 0.02 μM
5 mM Glucose	0.27 ± 0.03 μM
10 mM Glucose	0.54 ± 0.09 μM
20 mM Glucose	0.66 ± 0.07 μM

Table 2. Effect of [Substrate] on K_d of the high affinity binding sites of Glucokinase

4. Magnesium and gluconeogenesis

Gluconeogenesis is the process of glucose synthesis from non-carbohydrate precursors. Phosphoenolpyruvate Carboxy kinase (PEPCK), fructose1,6-bisphosphatase (F1,6BP), pyruvate carboxylase and glucose-6-phosphatase (G6Pase),catalyze irreversible reactions in the pathway and have lower activities compared to the other enzymes in the pathway and are thus considered rate limiting for glucose synthesis. Experiments by McNeill et al, [70] suggest that magnesium deficiency alters PEPCK by affecting secretion of pancreatic hormones. Of these four enzymes, $Mg^{2+}$is required by three, that is, pyruvate carboxylase, PEPCK, and F1, 6BP reactions. Though hormones such as insulin, glucagon, glucocorticoids and epinephrine influence the key enzyme activities of gluconeogenic enzymes, Mg^{2+}plays a role in the secretion of all these hormones [70]. Thus in Mg^{2+}deficiency, enzyme activities may change, as a result of altered circulating levels of one or more hormones. In this study like in earlier studies, an increase in PEPCK activity was observed in magnesium deficient rats making Mg^{2+}deficiency a possible contributing factor to the maintenance of low insulin levels an increased PEPCK in diabetes [70].

5. Conclusion

In the last two decades, our understanding of the importance of Mg^{2+}ions for numerous cell and body functions has increased significantly. The initial experimental evidence has been corroborated to a significant extent in clinical conditions such as diabetes, alcoholism, and dysendocrinopathies.

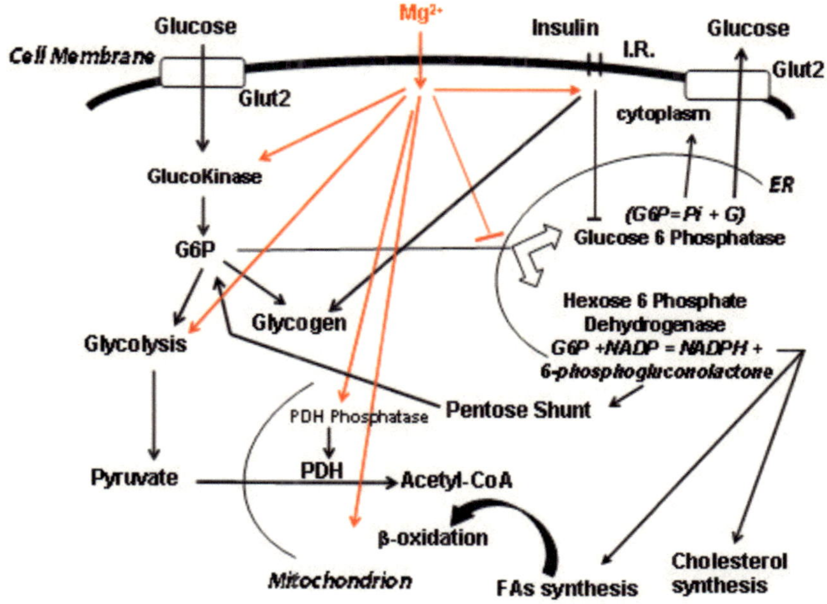

Figure 2. Graphic representations of the different glucose-related functions controlled by Mg^{2+}in the hepatocyte.`

In the case of liver cells, we have moved from the initial observation that $Mg^{2+}$is abundantly represented within the hepatocyte as a whole to the notion that the cation's homeostasis is controlled by hormones, which promotes the movement of Mg^{2+}in-and-out of the cell membrane to support and regulate specific liver metabolic functions. The observation that $Mg^{2+}$is highly compartmentalized within cellular compartments and organelles support the notion that the cation plays a key role in regulating enzymes, channel activities, and metabolic processes within each of these organelles. Figure 2 recapitulates the relevance of $Mg^{2+}$for the regulation of glucose homeostasis and bioenergetics within the hepatocyte. In the cytoplasm, Mg^{2+}regulates glucokinase and glycolytic enzymes but also ATP utilization. In the mtiochondria, Mg^{2+}regulates mitochondrial dehydrogenases and pyruvate dehydrogenase by promoting the activity of the pyruvate dehydrogenase phosphatase, responsible for dephosphorylating the enzyme to its active conformation. In the endoplasmic reticulum (ER), Mg^{2+}regulates protein synthesis and the entry of glucose 6 phosphate (G6P), the limiting step for the utilization of this substrate by the glucose 6-phosphatase (G6Pase) and the hexose 6-phosphate dehydrogenase (H6PD), the reticular variant of the cytosolic glucose 6 phosphate dehydrogenase (G6PD). The oxidation of G6P by the H6PD generates high levels of NADPH within the ER lumen to be used for other metabolic processes within the organelle and in the rest of the cell, including fatty acid synthesis and cholesterol synthesis. Far from being complete, the picture is a dynamic scenario in need to further clarification and study in the years to come.

Author details

Chesinta Voma[1,2] and Andrea M.P. Romani[1*]

*Address all correspondence to: amr5@po.cwru.edu

1 Department of Physiology and Biophysics, School of Medicine, Case Western Reserve University, Cleveland, OH, USA

2 Department of Clinical Chemistry, Cleveland State University, Cleveland, OH, USA

References

[1] Hoganson DM, Prior HI, Vacanti JP. Tissue Engineering and Organ Structure: A Vascularized Approach to liver and lung. Pediatric Research. 2008;63(5): 520-526

[2] Crawford JM. The liver and Biliary Tract. In: Robbins Pathologic Basis of Disease (Cotran RS, Kumar V, Collins J eds.), W.B. Saunders Company, Philadelphia, PA, 1999 pp 845-901

[3] Jungermann K, Katz N. Functional hepatocellular heterogeneity. Hepatology 1982;2: 385-395

[4] Jungermann K, Katz N. Functional specialization of different hepatocyte populations. Physiol Rev 1989;69: 708-764

[5] LeCluyse EL, Audus KL, Hochman JH. Formation of extensive canalicular networks by rat hepatocytes cultured in collagen-sandwich configuration. Am J Physiol 1994; 266:C1764-C1774

[6] Robey, RB, Hay N. Mitochondrial hexokinases, novel mediators of the antiapoptotic effects of growth factors and Akt. Oncogene 2006;25(34): 4683–4696

[7] Bánhegyi G, Benedetti A, Fulceri R, Senesi S. Cooperativity between 11beta-hydroxysteroid dehydrogenase type 1 and hexose-6-phosphate dehydrogenase in the lumen of the endoplasmic reticulum. J Biol Chem. 2004;279(26):27017-27021

[8] Berteloot A, Vidal H, van de Werve G. Rapid kinetics of liver microsomal glucose-6-phosphatase. Evidence for tight-coupling between glucose-6-phosphate transport and phosphohydrolase activity. J Biol Chem 1991;266: 5497–5507.

[9] Foster JD, Nordlie RC. The biochemistry and molecular biology of the glucose-6-phosphatase system. Exp Biol Med 2002;227:601–608

[10] Banhegy G, Marcolongo P, Fulceri R, Hinds C, Burchell A, Benedetti A. Demonstration of a metabolically active glucose-6-phosphate pool in the lumen of liver microsomal vesicles. J Biol Chem 1997;272:13584–13590.

[11] St-Denis J-F, Berteloot A, Vidal AH, Annabi B, van de Werve G. Glucose transport and glucose 6-phosphate hydrolysis in intact rat liver microsomes. J Biol Chem 1995; 270:21092–21097.

[12] Jungermann K, Heilbronn R, Katz N, Sasse D. The glucose/glucose-6-phosphate cycle in periportal and perivenous zone of rat liver. Eur J biochem 1982;123:479-436.

[13] Romani A, Fulceri R, Pompella A, Benedetti A. MgATP-dependent, glucose 6-phosphate-stimulated liver microsomal Ca^{2+}accumulation: difference between rough and smooth microsomes. Arch Biochem Biophys 1988;266(1):1-9.

[14] Fulceri R, Bellomo G, Gamberucci A, Romani A, Benedetti A. Physiological concentrations of inorganic phosphate affect MgATP-dependent Ca^{2+}storage and inositol trisphosphate-induced Ca^{2+}efflux in microsomal vesicles from non-hepatic cells. Biochem J 1993;289(Pt 1):299-306.

[15] Száraz P, Bánhegyi G, Benedetti A. Altered redox state of luminal pyridine nucleotides facilitates the sensitivity towards oxidative injury and leads to endoplasmic reticulum stress dependent autophagy in HepG2 cells. Int J Biochem Cell Biol 2010;42(1): 157-166

[16] He L, Cao J, Meng S, Ma A, Radovick S, Wondeisford FE. Activation of basal gluconeogenesis by coactivator p300 maintains hepatic glycogen storage. Mol Endocrino. 2013:27(8):1322-1332.

[17] http://www.whfoods.com

[18] http://bestpractices.bmj.com/best-pratice/monograph/1137.html

[19] Alfrey AC, Miller NL, Trow R. Effect of age and magnesium depletion on bone magnesium pools in rats. J Clin Invest 1974;54:1074-1081.

[20] Rude KK, Olerich M. Magnesium deficiency: possible role in osteoporosis associated with gluten-sensitive enteropathy. Osteoporos Int 1996;6:453-461.

[21] Romani A, Scarpa A. Regulation of cell magnesium. Arch Biochem Biophys 1992;298(1): 1-12

[22] Scarpa A, Brinley FJ. In situ measurements of cytosolic free magnesium ions. Fed Proc. 1981;40(12): 2646-2652

[23] Romani AM. Magnesium homeostasis in mammalian cells Met Ions Life Sci 2013;12:69-118

[24] Lüthi D, Günzel D, McGuigan JA. Mg-ATP binding: its modification by spermine, the relevance to cytosolic Mg^{2+}buffering, changes in the intracellular ionized

Mg^{2+}concentration and the estimation of $Mg^{2+}$by 31P-NMR. Exp Physiol 1999; 84(2): 231-52

[25] Cowan JA. Structural and catalytic chemistry of magnesium-dependent enzymes. Biometals 2002;15: 225-235.

[26] Garfinkle L, Garfinkle D. Magnesium regulation of the glycolytic pathway and the enzymes involved. Magnesium 1985;4(2-3):60-72.

[27] Volpe P, Alderson-Lang BH, Nickols GA. Regulation of inositol 1,4,5-trisphosphate-induced Ca^{2+}release. I. Effect of Mg^{2+}.Am. J. Physiol 1990; 258:C1077-C1085.

[28] Rubin H. Central roles of $Mg^{2+}$and $MgATP^{2-}$in the regulation of protein synthesis and cell proliferation: significance for neoplastic transformation. Adv Cancer Res 2005;93:1-58

[29] Barfell A, Crumbly A, Romani A. Enhanced glucose 6-phosphatase activity in liver of rats exposed to Mg^{2+}-deficient diet. Arch Biochem Biophys 2011;509(2):157-163.

[30] Gunther T. Functional compartmentation of intracellular magnesium. Magnesium 1986; 5:53-59.

[31] Kolisek M, Nestler A, Vormann J, Schweigel-Rontgen M. Human gene SLC41A1 encodes for the Na^{+}/Mg^{2+}exchanger. Am J Physiol. 2012, 302, C318-C326.

[32] Romani A. Cellular magnesium homeostasis. Arch. Biochem Biophys 2011;512:1-23.

[33] Romani A, Dowell E, Scarpa A. Cyclic-AMP-induced magnesium release from rat liver hepatocytes, permeabilized hepatocytes, and isolated mitochondria. J Biol Chem 1991;266(36): 24376-24384.

[34] Cefaratti C, Ruse C. Protein kinase A dependent phosphorylation activates Mg^{2+}efflux in the basolateral region of the liver. Mol Cell Biochem 2007;297(1-2): 209-214

[35] Mishra R, Rao V, Ta R, Shobeiri N, Hill CE. Mg^{2+}-and MgATP-inhibited and Ca^{2+}/calmodulin-sensitive TRPM7-like current in hepatoma and hepatocytes. Am J Physiol 2009; 297(4):G687-G694.

[36] Cao G, Thébault S, van der Wijst J, van der Kemp A, Lasonder E, Bindels RJ, Hoenderop JG. RACK1 inhibits TRPM6 activity via phosphorylation of the fused alpha-kinase domain. Curr Biol 2008;18(3):168-176.

[37] Romani A. In Physiology of Magnesium Homeostasis (Vink R, Nechifor M eds.) 2011, Univ. of Adelaide Publishing Co., Adelaide, Australia.

[38] Alexander RT, Hoenderop JG, Bindels RJ. Molecular determinants of magnesium homeostasis: insights from human disease.J. Am. Soc. Nephrol. 2008, 19, 1451-1458.

[39] Touyz RM, He Y, Montezano ACI, Yao G, Chubanov V, Gudemann T, Callera GE. Differential regulation of transient receptor potential melastatin 6 and 7 cation chan-

nels by ANG II in vascular smooth muscle cells from spontaneously hypertensive rats. Am J Physiol 2006;290:R73-R78.

[40] Fagan TE, Romani A. Activation of Na^+-and Ca^{2+}-dependent Mg^{2+}extrusion by alpha$_1$- and beta-adrenergic agonists in rat liver cells. Am J Physiol 2000;279:G943-G950

[41] Fagan TE, Romani A. alpha$_1$-Adrenoceptor-induced Mg^{2+}extrusion from rat hepatocytes occurs via Na^+-dependent transport mechanism. Am J Physiol 2001;280(6):G1145-G1156.

[42] Cefaratti C, Romani A, Scarpa A. Differential localization and operation of distinct Mg^{2+}transporters in apical and basolateral sides of rat liver plasma membranes. J Biol Chem 2000;275(6):3772-3780.

[43] Keenan D, Romani A, Scarpa A.Regulation of Mg^{2+}homeostasss by insulin in perfused rat livers and isolated hepatocytes. FEBS Lett 1996;395(2-3):241-244.

[44] Romani A, Marfella C, Scarpa A. Hormonal stimulation of Mg^{2+}uptake in hepatocytes. Regulation by plasma membrane and intracellular organelles. J Biol Chem 1993;268(21):15489-95.

[45] Maguire ME. Hormone-sensitive magnesium transport and magnesium regulation of adenylate cyclase. TIPS 1984:73-77.

[46] Romani AM. Magnesium homeostasis in mammalian cells. Front Biosci 2007;12:308-331.

[47] Ferreira A, Rivera A, Romero JR. Na^+/Mg^{2+}exchange is functionally coupled to the insulin receptor. J Cell Physiol. 2004;199(3):434-40.

[48] Romani A, Scarpa A. Hormonal control of Mg^{2+}transport in the heart. Nature 1990;346:841-844.

[49] Romani A, Scarpa A. Norepinephrine evokes a marked Mg^{2+}efflux from liver cells. FEBS Lett. 1990; 269(1);37-40.

[50] Piskacek M, Zotova L, Zsurka G, Schweyen RJ. Conditional knockdown of hMRS2 results in loss of mitochondrial Mg^{2+}uptake and cell death. J Cell Mol Med 2009;13(4): 693-700

[51] Gaussin V, Gailly P, Gillis J-M, Hue L. Fructose-induced increase in intracellular free Mg^{2+}ion concentration in rat hepatocytes: relation with the enzymes of glycogen metabolism. Biochem J 1997; 326:823-827.

[52] Dalal P, Romani A. Adenosine triphosphate depletion by cyanide results in a Na^+-dependent Mg^{2+}extrusion from liver cells. Metabolism 2010; 59:1663-1671.

[53] Fagan TE, Cefaratti C, Romani A. Streptozotocin-induced diabetes impairs Mg^{2+}homeostasis and uptake in rat liver cells. Am J Physiol 2004;286(2):E184-E193.

[54] Suarez A, Pulido N, Casla A, Casanova B, Arrieta FJ, Rovira A. Impaired Tyrosine-Kinase Activity of Muscle Insulin Receptors from Hypomagnesaemic Rats. Diabetologia 1995;38: 1262-1270.

[55] Cheng Z, Guo1 S, Copps K, Dong X, Kollipara R, Rodgers JT, Depinho RA, Puigserver P, White MF. Foxo1 integrates insulin signaling with mitochondrial function in the liver. Nature Medicine 2009;15:1307-1311.

[56] Alhadeff JA, Wolfe S. Characterization of Human Liver (4-Methylumbelliferyl-α-D-N-Acetylneuraminic Acid) Neuraminidase Activity. Int. J. Biochem 1981;13:975-980.

[57] Dribi L, Seyrantepe V, Fougerat A, Pan X, Bonneil E, Thibault P, Moreau A, Mitchell GA, Heveker N, Cairo CW, Issad T, Hinek A, Pshezheetsky AV. Positive Regulation of Insulin Signaling by Neuraminidase 1. Diabetes 2013; 62:2338-2346.

[58] Torres LM, Younger J, Romani A. Role of glucose in modulating Mg^{2+}homeostasis in liver cells from starved rats. Am. J. Physiol. 2005; 288(2) G195-G206.

[59] Barbagallo M, Dominguez LJ. Magnesium metabolism in type 2 diabetes mellitus, metabolic syndrome and insulin resistance.Arch Biochem. Biophys. 2007;458(1): 40-47

[60] Nadler J, Scott S. Evidence that pioglitazone increases intracellular free magnesium concentration in freshly isolated rat adipocytes. Biochem. Biophys, Res. Commun 1994; 202:416-421

[61] Guerrero-Romero F, Rodriguez-Moran M. Complementary therapies for diabetes: the case for chromium, magnesium, and antioxidants. Arch Med Res. 2005:36(3):250-257

[62] Cefaratti C, McKinnis A, Romani A. Altered Mg^{2+}transport across liver plasma membrane from streptozotocin-treated rats. Mol Cell Biochem 2004;262(1-2):145-54.

[63] Romani AM, Matthews VD, Scarpa A. Parallel stimulation of glucose and Mg^{2+}accumulation by insulin in rat hearts and cardiac ventricular myocytes. Circ Res 2000;86(3):326-33.

[64] Rude RK. Magnesium Defieciency: A Cause of Heterogenous Disease in Humans. J Bone Mineral Res 1998;13(4): 749-758.

[65] Romani AM. Magnesium Homeostasis and alcohol consumption. Magnesium Res 2008;21(4):197-204.

[66] Niemeyer H, Cardenas ML, Rabajille E, Ureta T, Clark-Turri, Penaranda J. Sigmoidal Kinetics of glucokinase. Enzyme 1975; 20:321-333.

[67] Storer AC, Cornish-Bowden A. Kinetics of rat-liver glucokinase: co-operative interactions with glucose at physiologically significant concentrations. Biochemical J 1976; 159:7-14.

http://dx.doi.org/10.5772/57564

[68] Agius L, Peak M, Newgard CB, Gomez-Foix AM, Guinovart JJ. Evidence for a Role of Glucose–induced Translocation of Glucokinase in the control of Hepatic Glycogen Synthesis. J Biol Chem 1996; 271(48):30479-30486.

[69] Agius L, Peak M, Schaftingen EV. The regulatory protein of glucokinase binds to the hepatocyte matrix, but unlike glucokinase does not translocate during substrate stimulation. Biochem J 1995; 309, 711-713.

[70] McNeill DA, Herbein JH, Ritchey SJ. Hepatic Gluconeogenic enzymes, plasma insulin and glucagon response to magnesium deficiency and fasting. J Nutr 1982; 112(4): 736-743.

Chapter 5

Glycemia and Memory

M.O. Welcome and V.A. Pereverzev

Additional information is available at the end of the chapter

http://dx.doi.org/10.5772/58241

1. Introduction

One of the major functions of brain cells (neurons) is to receive, store, and participate in information retrieval – an important process for the successful daily activities of humans [1-3]. This function of neurons is termed 'memory' [1, 4, 5]. The present understanding of memory function is the product of the pioneering work of the German scientist Hermann Ebbinghaus [5]. Research suggests that many factors (both endogenous and exogenous) could affect memory function [6-8]. However, the effect of glucose on memory function remains extremely significant for the following reasons [9-12]. First, glucose is the vital energy substrate for neuronal functions [13, 14]. Second, inadequate level of glucose in the blood has been associated with a decrease in memory function [15]. Third, disorders in glucose metabolism have been related to various aspects of memory disorders [8, 16]. Furthermore, metabolic products of glucose in neurons themselves participate in one or more stages of memory formation [17-20]. Notwithstanding the significant accumulation of research data in last decades on the relationship between glycemia and neuronal functions [11, 12, 21], the mechanisms of how glucose affect memory functions remains entirely not understood. In this chapter, we shall examine the possible mechanisms and processes involved in the glucose regulation of memory function. We shall elaborate on the effect of glucose on the major processes of memory functions, precisely on the formation and retrieval of "neural data" – memory.

2. Memory as an integral function of neurons

More than 90% of human activities are dependent on higher integrative brain functions – a major subdivision, which is the topic of our discussion in the chapter. The higher integrative brain functions are the driving force during physical work. This is because the brain is the "chief" that directs resources for the successful completion of the task. Successful activities of humans are largely dependent on memory function [22]. This function of neurons becomes vividly indispensable in situations involving its disorder. Memory is that function of neurons that involve storage and retrieval of information [22]. Some researchers have argued "forgetting" as an important aspect of memory function [23, 24]. This is partly because without forgetting, some new information might hardly go into storage. Hence, there are theories of forgetting – the most known ones are the single-trace fragility theory, decay theory, retrieval failure, interference theory, repression, consolidation theory [22]. Generally, several concepts/theories/models/hypotheses have been used to explain memory function of neurons [22, 25-27]. However, with steady scientific progress it is becoming clearer that none of these gives a complete, and precise definition of memory. In this regard, we shall also discuss briefly on the modern concepts of memory function of neurons in relation to cerebral glucose metabolism.

3. Factors that affect memory: Scanning for glucose's role

Several factors affect memory functions, and they can either be endogenous or exogenous. Generally, the widely known substances/factors include narcotics, some prescription drugs, alcohol, some biomolecules (most notably glucose, fatty acids, amino acids), environmental factors, genetic and epigenetic factors [6-8, 21, 28]. Among the biomolecules that affect memory formation and retrieval, glucose is widely known and well-studied molecule. Glucose is the main substrate for memory formation and retrieval. Glucose not only provides the energy for memory formation and retrieval, but also, is involved in providing the necessary subunits or components for the formation of various neural components of the "neural data" – memory [9, 11, 12, 14, 21, 29, 30].

4. Glycemia: A key regulating factor for memory formation and retrieval

Decades of research have shown that a change in the glycemic level leads to a corresponding change in memory function of the brain [21, 29-41]. For example, decrease in blood glucose below the set point is reported to negatively affect memory function [9, 21, 29, 30]. Glycemia affect both memory formation and retrieval [9, 29].

Results of several studies have observed an inverted-U shaped dose-response relationship between glucose load and memory [31-34]. Recent study has shown that the optimum dose of glucose memory enhancement may differ under conditions of depleted glucose resources, and has other peculiarities [21].

Several controversies in the glucose memory facilitation effect remain. While some previous studies reported a "no effect relationship" between glucose and memory function [35, 36], others confirm this dose-response relationship [9, 31, 37, 38]. Researchers have suggested that this relationship is extremely dependent on the type of cognitive/memory task [39, 40].

Modulating factors of the glucose memory facilitation effect include physiological state (body mass index etc.), glucose dose, types of cognitive tasks used and cognitive demand [9, 39]. These factors are the possible sources of variance in the glucose facilitation of memory. Owen and colleagues (2008) investigated the dose response relationship of the glucose memory facilitation effect at glucose dosages of 0, 15, 25, 50 and 60 g [9]. They also examined the interactions between length of fasting interval (2 hours versus 12 hours) and the optimum dose of glucose. Their results revealed glucose facilitation of spatial working memory and verbal declarative memory following 25 g glucose. Furthermore, they observed that glucose memory facilitation effect is dependent on the following: the greater the length of fasting, the greater the glucose dose needed to facilitate memory [9]. So, at overnight fast (approximately 12 hours) the higher dose of glucose (i.e. 60 g) was needed to facilitate memory, whereas the lower dose (25 g) enhanced working memory performance following a 2 hour fast [9].

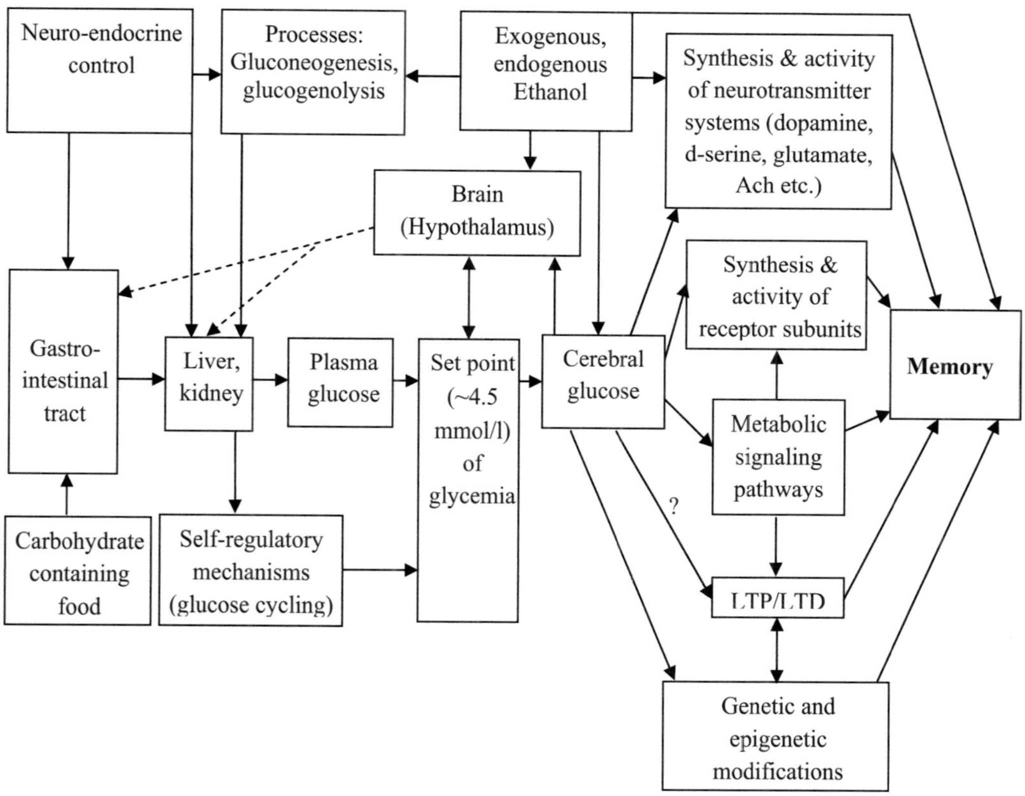

Figure 1. Comprehensive model of glucose memory facilitation

The mechanisms responsible for memory formation and retrieval are in constant perturbations of several factors (which might be competing factors, endogenous or exogenous in nature). The processes and mechanisms that ensure memory formation are the synthesis and activity of neurotransmitters (dopamine, d-serine, glutamate, acetylcholine etc), and receptor subunit systems; metabolic signaling pathways; LTP/LTD (long-term potentiation/ long-term depression); genetic and epigenetic modifications. (Memory retrieval might involve the same systems and processes, but with different mechanisms). Both memory formation and retrieval involve other brain functions, including attention. The systems and processes earlier stated are affected by cerebral glucose, which can serve as a substrate or produce intermediate substrates for some stages of their syntheses. The cerebral glucose content is dependent on the plasma glucose, both of which are under constant regulation by the brain (hypothalamus), some internal organs (liver, kidney). The blood glucose is constantly regulated, also by the effect of the neuro-endocrine control on the gastrointestinal tract, organs (such as the liver and kidney), as well as the effect of the hypothalamus on these organs. The processes that are regulated in these organs by the higher regulatory centres (e.g. hypothalamus) are food intake, gluconeogenesis, glycogenolysis, glucose cycling – to ensure normal glycemic allostasis. These higher control centres, and the memory function are under constant pressure from modulating factors such as exogenous (e.g. environmental, ethanol), endogenous (ethanol, some physiological indices) – might affect the resultant effect of glucose on memory function. Alcohol actions [42-45] as represented on the model are one of a bi-directional effect of summation, meaning that alcohol affects memory, as well as glucose regulatory systems. The receptor systems of the brain could be modulated by both alcohol and glucose [46, 47]. Alcohol is a psychotic substance in widespread usage in the world. Importantly, this substance is also produced in vivo during biochemical reactions in an organism (including humans). In certain circumstances (varying physiological state, for instance during pregnancy, disease states), the level of endogenous ethanol produced significantly increases. This increase might have a protective effect, but the reason or mechanism on the general role of the increase in endogenous concentration ethanol is not fully known. Ethanol affects some neurotransmitters and receptor systems. Ethanol acts on ionotropic, metabotropic G-protein receptor, potassium ion channels [48-50]. Ethanol acts on metabotropic receptors of mGluR5, mGluR2/3, mGluR1 [51-53]. These metabotropic receptors (mGluR3 of the prefrontal cortex) have been also implicated in cognitive disorders in especially alcoholics [54]. mGluR5 and mGluR1 receptors have been recently implicated in cognition [53]. Ethanol causes hypoglycemia [43, 55]. Besides, it is reported that alcohol causes disorders in the expression of several genes, although the mechanisms remain not quite clear [56].

Glucose plays a pivotal role in memory and might enhance LTP/LTD [57] as hypoglycemia is associated with deficits in memory, and learning [58, 59]. Apart from producing ATP for neural energy, other substances may be synthesized from glucose that affects neuronal activity and functions (including memory) [60-62]. For example, it is known that d-serine (maybe synthesized from glucose molecule) affects LTP, synaptic plasticity, enhance information retrieval [60-64]. Hypoglycemia is associated with both d-serine and NO release aimed at enhancing LTP [58]. These substances can also regulate neuronal transcription factors [65]. A vast number of these signaling pathways, neurotransmitter and receptor systems, and are dependent on the activity level of neurons, and activity dependent transcriptions – activators and suppressor [66, 67]. Other brain cells (especially astrocytes) can modulate neuronal activity through various mechanisms, involving NMDA, d-serine, Ca2+, ATP, glutamate. Hence, these brain cells, which are affected by ethanol, might exert their resultant effect on neurons through astroglial linkages [68, 69].

5. Mechanisms of glucose effect on memory

While several studies have noted that glucose is a critical factor for memory function, what is not exactly clear is whether the effect is a direct or indirect one. In this section, we shall be mainly concerned with the mechanisms and processes of how glucose affects memory. Pertinent literature and latest developments in the field will be reviewed. It will be necessary to have in mind that memory function (formation and retrieval of neural data) is overlapped or is connected with other brain functions such as perception, attention etc. Therefore, glucose is a vital regulating factor for other brain functions. We shall consider the various views, concepts and models of how glucose affects memory function, and provide a comprehensive model of glucose memory facilitation effect (Figure 1).

5.1. Conceptual model of glucose memory facilitation

Smith and colleagues (2011) suggested a conceptual model of glucose facilitation of memory. Their neurocognitive model stipulates that glucose or acute stress/emotional arousal increases the concentration of circulating glucose in the periphery, and subsequently, the central nervous system. This increase in glucose exerts its effects on insulin, acetylcholine (Ach) synthesis and/or K_{ATP} channel function which subsequently leads to memory enhancement. Research has confirmed that there is specific cognitive domain that is most amenable to the glucose memory facilitation effect. The domain is episodic memory [41].

5.2. Comprehensive model of glucose memory facilitation

Memory formation or retrieval involves the synthesis of many biomolecules related to glucose metabolism [41, 70-73]. Glucose memory facilitation effect is a complex phenomenon comprising of several players including organs/systems of glucose metabolism, several competing factors, both genetic and epigenetic [42, 46, 72, 74]. Based on available data, here we propose a comprehensive model of glucose memory facilitation.

5.2.1. Neurotransmitter systems

Several neurotransmitter systems have been implicated in memory function. Here, we shall briefly consider a few of the principal neurotransmitter systems involved in memory function. The literatures report significant role of dopaminergic, glutamatergic, serotonergic, cholinergic, and noradrenergic systems in memory function [75-78]. We shall consider d-serine involvement in memory formation owing to the fact that its main receptor – the NMDA receptor is one of the key receptors involved in long-term memory formation (as a result of its long-term potentiation effect). Long-term potentiation, as opposed to long-term depression is an integral process necessary for memory formation (especially long-term memory) [68, 69]. In fact, the NMDA receptor itself is implicated as one of the "alcohol receptors" [79]. Therefore, bi-directional effect of summation might occur through alcohol effect on neurotransmitter receptor systems, and glucose metabolism. The resultant effect is aggravation of memory dysfunction.

5.2.2. Metabolic signaling pathways

Since glucose is a metabolic product or must be involved in the cell's metabolic pathways before its usefulness is realized; therefore, it is necessary to assume that metabolic pathways, involving glucose molecule are those pathways crucial for memory formation or retrieval. Unfortunately, research in this aspect is scanty. A number of signaling pathways are involved in glucose metabolism, but there is no sufficient evidence on how they are associated with memory function [80]. The widely studied signaling pathways that have a relationship between glucose metabolism and memory functions [81, 82] include CREB pathway [83, 84], AMPK [85, 86], Notch signaling [87], mTOR pathway [88] etc. The mTOR pathway has been majorly implicated in both glucose and memory function. Importantly, it was reported that glucose specifically affects memory through this pathway [84, 88, 89].

5.2.3. Genetic and epigenetic regulation (activity dependent genes and epigenetic factors)

The enhancement of memory by glucose might be related partly to the functions of activity dependent genes [90, 91], as well as epigenetic modifications (DNA methylation and histone modifications) by glucose or its metabolites [10, 91-94].

Since epigenetic profile of the cells play crucial role in glucose metabolism and neuronal cell functions, here, we would suggest that the initial epigenetic data (program) of the involved cells responsible for glucose memory facilitation are partly important for the differences reported in the literature. Epigenetic mechanisms of glucose metabolism and memory functions are regulated by the activity of transcription factors [10, 95]. Due to the importance of glucose in the functioning of the CNS [96], this regulation may be modulated by glucose molecule itself. For example, the data of Li et al. (2010) indicate that glucose regulates gene transcription in the liver by increasing the level of ATP, hence inhibiting AMP-activated protein kinase and inducing hepatocyte nuclear factor 4alpha to stimulate cytochrome P450 7A1 gene transcription. Glucose also increases histone acetylation and decreases H3K9 methylation in the cytochrome P450 7A1 chromatin [97].

Recent experiments show that glucose is involved in the regulation of functions even at the progenitor cell level. Metabolism-sensing factors have recently been implicated in the regulation of neural stem cell fate through epigenetics modification [92, 98]. Hayakawa et al. (2013) reported that in embryonic stem cell population, glucose metabolite induces switching from the inactive state by Ogt-Sirt1 to the active state by Mgea5, p300, and CBP at the Hcrt gene locus [92]. The many pathways of glucose metabolism allows for the inclusion of its metabolic products into numerous cellular activities. For example, substrates of glucose metabolic pathways (acetyl-CoA, ATP, NAD+, glutamine, UDP-N-acetyl-glucosamine, N-acetyl-Dmannosamine etc.) are candidates of epigenetic modifications. Acetyl-CoA is a donor of histone acetylation. NAD+regulates Sirt1, a member of the sirtuin family, which functions as histone deacetylase and is also a metabolic sensor [92] (for review see Hayakawa et al. 2013). Epigenetic regulation by glucose or its metabolites affects memory functions and glucose metabolism itself through a shift in the cellular concentrations of critical metabolites implicated in higher integrative brain functions and metabolism.

A key mechanism for this epigenetic regulation is executed by the peripheral circadian oscillation [99]. However, importantly the peripheral clock and the central one could have some kind of metabolic associations. The concentration of NAD+/NADH plays critical link between metabolism and circadian rhythm [99]. Glucose and other metabolic substances may modulate the circadian rhythm by fluctuations in NAD+/NADH ratio. Compelling evidences now indicate that circadian misalignment could cause serious metabolic problems. In fact, transgenerational inheritance in metabolic alterations could be related to some mechanisms of epigenetic origin modulated by circadian clocks. Methylation of the leptin gene is associated with impaired glucose tolerance in the period of gestation [100]. This and many other discoveries on transgenerational inheritance represent substantial contribution to understanding the pathogenesis of diabetes, obesity in children [100-102].

Epigenetic regulations are not only affected by metabolites, but also body mass index, intrauterine environment, exercise, and other environmental factors [101].

It might be possible that epigenetic dysregulation of cerebral glucose metabolism is the result of cognitive impairment since glucose metabolism is controlled by epigenetic mechanisms and is also associated with cognition. Emerging evidences indicate that metabolic regulation (through epigenetic mechanisms) might be involved in memory function disorders. Reports show that a major pathogenesis of the CNS disorder such as Alzheimer's disease involves metabolic alterations, especially in glucose metabolism and associated hormonal or peptide signaling. Metabolic disorders in CNS pathologies are associated with brain insulin signaling. For example, a substantial quantity of insulin receptors is located in the hippocampus (a brain region which is basically concerned with the acquisition, consolidation and recall of new information) [103]. Impaired brain insulin signaling is implicated in cognitive impairment. Moreover, cognitive impairment is associated with diabetes and obesity, which are metabolic disorders [104]. De la Monte (2009) reported that in the initial stage of Alzheimer's disease, cerebral glucose metabolism is reduced by 45% and cerebral blood flow approximately by 18% [104]. Earlier, Arnáiz et al. (2001) reported that among twenty patients with mild cognitive impairment, impaired cerebral glucose metabolism and cognitive functioning were able to predict deterioration in mild cognitive impairment [105]. Mild cognitive impairment is an important indicator of the development of Alzheimer's disease. Notably, impairment in cerebral glucose metabolism was even a better predictor (75%) compared to neurospcyhological tests (65%) widely used in the assessment of cognitive impairment [105]. The authors further concluded that measures of temporoparietal cerebral metabolism and visuospatial function may aid in predicting the evolution to Alzheimer's disease for patients with mild cognitive impairment [105].

These data are very important especially when we consider the increasing prevalence of cognitive disorders. For instance, it is estimated that in 2030 years, the cases of Alzheimer's disease in relation to 2012 will double (35.6 million). No doubts, research in this direction is exceedingly necessary [106]. Previously other authors have also reported that impairment in cerebral glucose metabolism is associated with decline in cognition and memory functions. Schapiro et al (1988) studied the rate of cerebral metabolism for glucose with positron emission tomography and [18F]2-fluoro-2-deoxy-D-glucose in a 47 year-old man with trisomy 21 Down's syndrome and Alzheimer related dementia, and reported poorer general intelligence, visuospatial ability, language, and memory function compared with younger (19-33 years) patients with Down's syndrome [107]. Cerebral metabolism for glucose in the older patient was 28% less than in the younger patients. Besides, hypometabolism was reported in the parietal and temporal lobes of the brain cortices. Importantly, the study of Schapiro et al (1988) was probably one of the most comprehensive investigations to show the association between different diseases involving CNS disorder and their relationship with cerebral glucose metabolism [107]. Approximately a decade after Schapiro et al.'s (1988) work [107], Pietrini et al. (1997) reported another predictor method for Alzheimer's disease risk prior to dementia in patients with Down's syndrome who were above 40 years (mean of 50 years) of age [108]. Pietrini, et al. (1997) confirmed their hypothesis that despite normal cerebral glucose metabolism at rest, an audiovisual stimulation (was used as a stress test) revealed abnormalities in cerebral glucose metabolism before the development of dementia in the parietal and temporal cortices which represent most vulnerable regions to Alzheimer's disease [108].

These CNS pathologies are now believed to be regulated by epigenetic mechanisms [109] and could have pretty good correlations with epigenetic mechanisms of cerebral glucose metabolism. Other CNS pathologies involving cognitive impairments such as epilepsy [110], schizophrenia [111, 112], Parkinson's disease [113], multiple sclerosis [114] had been associated with disturbances in glucose metabolism.

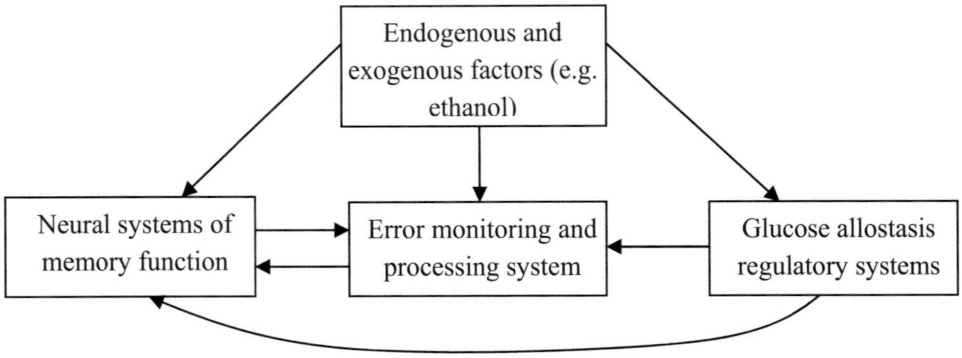

Figure 2. Interacting system (comprising of memory function, error monitoring and processing system, and modulators) of the reciprocability of neural systems of memory and the error monitoring and processing system. The modulators between the two reciprocals are glucose, other endogenous and exogenous substances/factors. N/B: Glucose can be an endogenous, as well as an exogenous factor; exogenous sources include per os administration of glucose, etc.; endogenous sources include gluconeogenetic production of glucose molecules, etc.

6. Glucose error commission depression effect: Cue to an overlapping bridge of neural error systems, memory and glucose metabolism?

Our data and those of other authors show strong negative relations between glycemia and error commission. Whether this is due to the effect of glucose on memory or neural systems of error commission, is what is not exactly clear (see figure 2). There are no precise borders between the brain regions responsible for memory and error commission. Therefore, it is possible that the effect of glucose on error commission could be the resultant effect on the chief brain regions for memory function. Neural systems (or regions) of memory implicated in error commission have been linked to brain regions also involved in some aspects of memory function [115-117]. The brain systems concerned with error commission are referred to the error monitoring and processing system. The major regions of the brain concerned with error commission are the anterior cingulate cortex, basal ganglia, prefrontal cortex. These brain regions (especially the prefrontal cortex) are also implicated in memory function [45, 115, 117].

7. Effect of alcohol on glycemia and memory: More than just a bi-directional modulating effect

Alcohol is the most prevalent psychotic substance in the world. While alcohol affects glucose metabolism, memory also remains one of the most vulnerable functions of the brain that suffers from the negative effect of alcohol use [15, 16, 29, 30, 44, 45, 118]. Hence, there is the need to examine its effect on memory function and glucose regulatory mechanisms. Here, we view alcohol as a positive modulating factor for memory (especially at endogenous concentration), and as a psychopathological substance at blood concentrations higher than the normal physiological level.

8. Conclusion

Glucose is the foremost energy substrate for neuronal functions (memory). It provides the energy bonds needed for the formation of memory and takes part in information retrieval from neural stores. Both glucose and its metabolites are involved in different stages of memory formation and retrieval. Several factors such as ethanol, some physiological indices, and other competing factors modulate the effect of glucose on memory function.

Author details

M.O. Welcome and V.A. Pereverzev

Belarusian State Medical University, Minsk, Belarus

References

[1] Sokolov EN. Brain Functions: Neuronal Mechanisms of Learning and Memory. Annu Rev Psychol 1977; 28: 85-112.

[2] Funahashi S. Neuronal mechanisms of executive control by the prefrontal cortex. Neurosci Res 2001; 39: 147 – 165.

[3] Parker BA, Polk DM, Rabdiya V, Meda SA, Anderson K, Hawkins KA, Pearlson GD, Thompson PD. Changes in Memory Function and Neuronal Activation Associated with Atorvastatin Therapy. Pharmacotherapy 2010;30(6):236e–240e.

[4] Endel T. Ebbinghaus's memory: What did he learn and remember? J Exp Psychol Learn Mem Cogn 1985; 11(3): 485-490.

[5] Ebbinghaus H. Memory: A contribution to experimental psychology. New York: Dover; 1964/original work published in 1885.

[6] Win-Shwe TT, Ohtani S, Ushiyama A, Fujimaki H, Kunugita N. Can intermediate-frequency magnetic fields affect memory function-related gene expressions in hippocampus of C57BL/6J mice? J Toxicol Sci 2013;38(2):169-76.

[7] Buffardi L. Factors affecting memory span in binary and octal responding. Am J Psychol 1972; 85 (3):377-391.

[8] Othman Z, Jamaluddin R, Alwi MNM, Ismail HC. Demographic And Clinical Factors Associated With Verbal Memory Performance In Patients With Schizophrenia In Hospital Universiti Sains Malaysia (HUSM), Malaysia. Asean J Psychiatr 2011;12 (2).

[9] Owen L, Sünram-Lea SI. Glucose facilitation of cognition: Factors responsible for variability in behavioural response. Appetite 2008; 50 (2-3): 564.

[10] Owen L, Sunram-Lea SI. Metabolic Agents that Enhance ATP can Improve Cognitive Functioning: A Review of the Evidence for Glucose, Oxygen, Pyruvate, Creatine, and L-Carnitine. Nutrients 2011; 3: 735-755.

[11] Sünram-Lea SI, Dewhurst SA, Foster JK. The effect of glucose administration on the recollection and familiarity components of recognition memory. Biol Psychol 2008;77(1):69-75.

[12] Korol DL, Gold PE. Glucose, memory, and aging. Am J Clin Nutr 1998;67(suppl): 764S–71S.

[13] Hoyland A, Dye L, Lawton CL. A systematic review of the effect of breakfast on the cognitive performance of children and adolescents. Nutr Res Rev 2009; 22:220-243.

[14] Owen L, Finnegan Y, Hu H, Scholey AB, Sünram-Lea SI. Glucose effects on long-term memory performance: duration and domain specificity. Psychopharmacology (Berl) 2010;211(2):131-40.

[15] Welcome MO, Pereverzeva EV, Pereverzev VA. Long-term disorders of cognitive functions in sober people who episodically use alcohol, role of functional hypoglycemia and insufficiency of gluconeogenesis. Vestnik Smolensk Med Acad 2011; 3: 2-20.

[16] Welcome MO, Razvodovsky YE, Pereverzeva EV, Pereverzev VA. State of cognitive functions of students-medics with different relationship to alcohol use. Minsk: Belarusian State Medical University Press; 2013.

[17] Hoyer S. memory function and brain glucose metabolism. Pharmacopsychiatry 2003; 36 (1):S62-S67.

[18] Riege WH, Metter EJ, Kuhl de, Phelps ME. Brain Glucose Metabolism and Memory Functions: Age Decrease in Factor Scores. J Gerontol 1985; 40(4): 459-467.

[19] Newcomer JW, Craft S, Fucetola R, Moldin SO, Selke Q, Paras L-U, Miller R. Glucose-Induced Increase in Memory Performance in Patients With Schizophrenia. Schizophrenia Bulletin 1999; 25(2):321-335.

[20] Qin M, Smith BC. Regionally selective decreases in cerebral glucose metabolism in a mouse model of phenylketonuria. J Inherit Metab Dis 2007;30(3):318-25.

[21] Owen L, Scholey A, Finnegan Y, Sünram-Lea SI. Response variability to glucose facilitation of cognitive enhancement. Br J Nutr 2013, In press.

[22] Baddeley A. Working Memory: Theories, Models, and Controversies. Annu Rev Psychol 2012;63:1–29.

[23] Wickelgren WA. Single-trace fragility theory of memory dynamics. Mem Cogn 1974; 2 (4): 775-780.

[24] Wixted JT. Analyzing the Empirical Course of Forgetting. J Exp Psychol Learn Mem Cogn 1990; 16 (5): 927-935.

[25] Chechile RA. Memory Hazard Functions: A Vehicle for Theory Development and Test. Psychol Rev 2006;113(1):31–56.

[26] Loflus GR. Consistency and Confoundings: Reply to Slamecka. J Exp Psychol Learn Mem Cogn 1985; 11 (4): 817-820.

[27] Saraswat V, Jagadeesan R, Michael M, von Praun C. A Theory of Memory Models. Proceedings of the 12th ACM SIGPLAN symposium on Principles and practice of parallel programming, ACM New York, NY, USA; 2007. p. 161 – 172.

[28] Bazan NG, Packard MG, Teather L, Allan G. Bioactive lipids in excitatory neurotransmission and neuronal plasticity. Neurochem Int 1997;30(2):225-31.

[29] Welcome MO, Razvodovsky YE, Pereverzeva EV, Pereverzev VA. The effect of blood glucose concentration on the error monitoring and processing system in alcohol users during intensive mental activities. Port Harcourt Med J 2011; 5 (3) 293-306.

[30] Welcome MO, Razvodovsky YE, Pereverzeva EV, Pereverzev VA. The error monitoring and processing system in alcohol use. IJCRIMPH. 2010; 2 (10): 318-336.

[31] Rodriguez WA, Horne CA, Padilla JL. Effects of glucose and fructose on recently reactivated and recently acquired memories. Prog Neuropsychopharmacol Biol Psychiatry 1999;23(7):1285-317.

[32] Baldi E, Bucherelli C. The inverted "U-shaped" dose-effect relationships in learning and memory: modulation of arousal and consolidation. Nonlinear Biol Toxicol Med 2005;3: 9–21.

[33] McEwen BS, Sapolsky RM. Stress and cognitive function. Curr Opin Neurobiol 1995; 5(2):205-216.

[34] Flint Jr W. Emotional Arousal, Blood Glucose Levels, and Memory Modulation: Three Laboratory Exercises in Cognitive Neuroscience. J Undergrad Neurosci Educ 2004, 3(1):A16 – A23.

[35] Azari NP. Effects of glucose on memory processes in young adults. Psychopharmacology (Berl) 1991;105(4):521-4.

[36] Gold PE, Vogt J, Hall JL. Glucose effects on memory: behavioral and pharmacological characteristics. Behav Neural Biol 1986;46(2):145-55.

[37] Rodriguez WA, Horne CA, Mondragon AN, Phelps DD. Comparable dose-response functions for the effects of glucose and fructose on memory. Behav Neural Biol 1994;61(2):162-9.

[38] Sünram-Lea SI, Owen L, Finnegan Y, Hu H. Dose-response investigation into glucose facilitation of memory performance and mood in healthy young adults. J Psychopharmacol 2011;25(8):1076-87.

[39] Sünram-Lea SI, Foster JK, Durlach P, Perez C. Investigation into the significance of task difficulty and divided allocation of resources on the glucose memory facilitation effect. Psychopharmacology (Berl) 2002;160(4):387-97.

[40] Foster JK, Lidder PG, Sünram SI. Glucose and memory: fractionation of enhancement effects? Psychopharmacology (Berl) 1998;137(3):259-70.

[41] Smith MA, Riby LM, van Eekelen JAM, Foster JK. Glucose enhancement of human memory: A comprehensive research review of the glucose memory facilitation effect. Neuroscience & Biobehavioral Rev 2011; 35(3): 770–783.

[42] Wickelgren WA. Alcoholic intoxication and memory storage dynamics. Mem Cognit 1975 ;3(4):385-9.

[43] De Galan BE, Schouwenberg BJ, Tack CJ, Smits P. Pathophysiology and management of recurrent hypoglycaemia and hypoglycaemia unawareness in diabetes. Neth J Med 2006; 64:269-279.

[44] Welcome MO. The state of higher integrative functions of the brain and level of glycemia in young adults who use alcoholic beverages. PhD thesis. Belarusian State Medical University; 2013.

[45] Welcome MO, Pereverzev VA. Basal Ganglia and the Error Monitoring and Processing System: How Alcohol Modulates the Error Monitoring and Processing Capacity of the Basal Ganglia (P). In: Barrios FA, Bauer C (ed.) Basal Ganglia – An Integrative View. Croatia: InTech; 2013. p. 65-86.

[46] Ungerer A, Mathis C, Mélan C. Are glutamate receptors specifically implicated in some forms of memory processes? Exp Brain Res 1998;123(1-2):45-51.

[47] Haltia LT, Rinne JO, Merisaari H, Maguire RP, Savontaus E, Helin S, Någren K, et al. Effects of intravenous glucose on dopaminergic function in the human brain in vivo. Synapse 2007; 61: 748 – 756.

[48] Cowen MS, Djouma E, Lawrence AJ. The Metabotropic Glutamate 5 Receptor Antagonist 3-[(2-Methyl-1, 3-thiazol-4-yl)ethynyl]-pyridine Reduces Ethanol Self-Administration in Multiple Strains of Alcohol-Preferring Rats and Regulates Olfactory Glutamatergic Systems. JPET 2005; 315:590–600.

[49] Bird MK, Lawrence AJ. Group I Metabotropic Glutamate Receptors: Involvement in Drug-Seeking and Drug-Induced Plasticity. Curr Mol Pharmacol 2009; 2: 83-94.

[50] Luscher C, Ungless MA. The mechanistic classification of addictive drugs. PLoS Med 2006; 3(11): e437. doi:10.1371/journal.pmed.0030437.

[51] Hodge CW, Miles MF, Sharko AC, Stevenson RA, Hillman JR, Lepoutre V, Besheer J, Schroeder JP. The mGluR5 antagonist MPEP selectivity inhibits the onset and maintenance of ethanol self-administration in mice. Psychopharmacology 2006;183: 429-438.

[52] Carta M, Mameli M, Valenzuela CF. Alcohol Potently Modulates Climbing Fiber3Purkinje Neuron Synapses: Role of Metabotropic Glutamate Receptors. J Neurosci 2006; 26(7):1906 –1912.

[53] Olive MF. Metabotropic glutamate receptor ligands as potential therapeutics for addiction. Curr Drug Abuse Rev 2009; 2(1): 83–989.

[54] Xia Y, Ma D, Hu J, Tang C, Wu Z, Liu L, Xin F. Effect of metabotropic glutamate receptor 3 genotype on N-acetylaspartate levels and neurocognition in non-smoking, active alcoholics. Behav Brain Functions 2012; 8:42.

[55] Krebs, H. A. and Perkins, J. R. The physiological role of liver alcohol dehydrogenase. Biochem J 1970; 118: 635–644.

[56] Pignataro L, Miller AN, Ma L, Midha S, Protiva P, Herrera DG, Harrison NL. Alcohol Regulates Gene Expression in Neurons via Activation of Heat Shock Factor 1. J Neurosci 2007; 27(47):12957–12966.

[57] Gault VA, Holscher C. Protease-resistant glucose-dependent insulinotropic polypeptide agonists facilitate hippocampal LTP and reverse the impairment of LTP induced by beta-amyloid. J Neurophysiol 2008; 99:1590-1595.

[58] Zorumski CF, Izumi Y. Modulation of LTP induction by NMDA receptor activation and nitric oxide release. Prog Brain Res 1998;118:173-82.

[59] Godfraind JM, Xu YZ. Two-deoxyglucose-induced long-term potentiation in slices of rat dentrate gyrus. Crit Rev Neurobiol 2006;18(1-2):37-48.

[60] Cui C, Grandison L, Noronha A. Neural-Immune Interactions in Brain Function and Alcohol Related Disorders. New York: Springer-Verlag; 2012.

[61] Wolosker H. D-serine regulation of NMDA receptor activity. Sci STKE 2006;2006(356):pe41.

[62] Rosenberg D, Kartvelishvily E, Shleper M, Klinker CMC, Bowser MT, Wolosker H. Neuronal release of D-serine: a physiological pathway controlling extracellular D-serine concentration. FASEB J 2010; 24: 2951–2961.

[63] Zhang Z, Gong N, Wang W, Xu L, Xu T-L. Bell-Shaped D-Serine Actions on Hippocampal Long-Term Depression and Spatial Memory Retrieval. Cerebral Cortex 2008;18:2391-2401.

[64] Zhuang Z, Yang B, Theus MH, Sick JT, Bethea JR, Sick TJ, Liebl DJ. EphrinBs regulate D-serine synthesis and release in astrocytes. J Neurosci 2010; 30(47): 16015–16024.

[65] Contestabile A. Regulation of transcription factors by nitric oxide in neurons and in neural-derived tumor cells. Prog Neurobiol 2008;84(4):317-28.

[66] West AE, Griffith EC, Greenberg ME. Regulation of transcription factors by neuronal activity. Nature Rev Neurosci 2002; 3: 921-931.

[67] Zhang J, Shapiro MS. Activity-Dependent Transcriptional Regulation of M-Type (Kv7) K+Channels by AKAP79/150-Mediated NFAT Actions. Neuron 2012; 76 (6): 1133-1146.

[68] Yang Y, Ge W, Chen Y, Zhang Z, Shen W, Wu C, Poo M, Duan S. Contribution of astrocytes to hippocampal long-term potentiation through release of D-serine. PNAS 2003; 100 (25):15194–15199.

[69] Henneberger C, Papouin T, Oliet SHR, Rusakov DA. Long-term potentiation depends on release of D-serine from astrocytes. Nature 2010; 463: 232-234.

[70] Herculano-Houzel S. Scaling of Brain Metabolism with a Fixed Energy Budget per Neuron: Implications for Neuronal Activity, Plasticity and Evolution. PLoS One 2011; 6(3): e17514. doi:10.1371/journal.pone.0017514.

[71] Nehlig A, Coles JA. Cellular pathways of energy metabolism in the brain: is glucose used by neurons or astrocytes? Glia 2007;55(12):1238-50.

[72] Jakoby P, Schmidt E, Ruminot I, Gutiérrez R, Barros LF, Deitmer JW. Higher Transport and Metabolism of Glucose in Astrocytes Compared with Neurons: A Multiphoton Study of Hippocampal and Cerebellar Tissue Slices. Cereb Cortex 2014;24(1): 222-31.

[73] Sibson NR. Stoichiometric coupling of brain glucose metabolism and glutamatergic neuronal activity. Proc Natl Acad Sci USA 1998; 95: 316 –321.

[74] Tsacopoulos M, Magistretti PJ. Metabolic Coupling between Glia and Neurons. J Neurosci 1996;76(3):877-885.

[75] Wenk G, Hughey D, Boundy V, Kim A, Walker L, Olton D. Neurotransmitters and memory: role of cholinergic, serotonergic, and noradrenergic systems. Behav Neurosci 1987;101(3):325-32.

[76] Shetty DN, Pathak SS. Correlation between plasma neurotransmitters and memory loss in pregnancy. J Reprod Med 2002;47(6):494-6.

[77] Dash PK, Moore AN, Kobori N, Runvan JD. Molecular activity underlying working memory. Learn Mem 2007; 14: 554-563.

[78] Berry JA, Cervantes-Sandoval I, Nicholas EP, Davis RL. Dopamine Is Required for Learning and Forgetting in Drosophila. Neuron 2012; 74 (3):530-542.

[79] Feyder M, Camp MC, Holmes A, Chen Y-C. Ethanol and NMDA Receptor Interactions: Implications for Pharmacotherapeutic Treatments. J Med Sci 2010;30(1): 003-010.

[80] Teperino R, Amann S, Bayer M, McGee SL, Loipetzberger A, Connor T, et al. Hedgehog Partial Agonism Drives Warburg-like Metabolism in Muscle and Brown Fat. Cell 2012; 151 (2): 414. doi: 10.1016/j.cell.2012.09.021.

[81] Graham NA, Tahmasian M, Koshli B, et al. Glucose deprivation activates a metabolic and signaling amplification loop leading to cell death. Mol Syst Biol 2012;8:589. doi: 10.1038/msb.2012.20.

[82] Summers SA, Yin VP, Whiteman EL, Garza LA, Cho H, Tuttle RL, Birnbaum MJ. Signaling Pathways Mediating Insulin-Stimulated Glucose Transport. Ann NY Acad Sci 1999; 892:169-186.

[83] Aonurm-Helm A, Zharkovsky T, Jürgenson M, Kalda A, Zharkovsky A. Dysregulated CREB signaling pathway in the brain of neural cell adhesion molecule (NCAM)-deficient mice. Brain Res 2008 3;1243:104-12.

[84] Simons AL, Orcutt KP, Madsen JM, Scarbrough PM, Spitz DR. The Role of Akt Pathway Signaling in Glucose Metabolism and Metabolic Oxidative Stress. In: Spitz DR et al. (eds.) Oxidative Stress in Cancer Biology and Therapy, Oxidative Stress in Applied Basic Research and Clinical Practice. LLC: Springer; 2012. p. 21-46.

[85] Potter WB, O'Riordan KJ, Barnett D, Osting SMK, Wagoner M, et al. Metabolic Regulation of Neuronal Plasticity by the Energy Sensor AMPK. PLoS One 2010; 5(2): e8996. doi:10.1371/journal.pone.0008996.

[86] Felipe BL. Metabolic signaling by lactate in the brain. Trends Neurosci 2013. 10.1016/j.tins.2013.04.002.

[87] Lasky JL, Wu H. Notch Signaling, Brain Development, and Human Disease. Pediatr Res 2005; 57: 104R–109R.

[88] Hoeffer CA, Klann E. mTOR Signaling: At the Crossroads of Plasticity, Memory, and Disease. Trends Neurosci 2010; 33(2): 67. doi:10.1016/j.tins.2009.11.003.

[89] Dash PK, Orsi SA, Moore AN. Spatial Memory Formation and Memory-Enhancing Effect of Glucose Involves Activation of the Tuberous Sclerosis Complex–Mammalian Target of Rapamycin Pathway. J Neurosci 2006; 26(31):8048–8056.

[90] Melzer P, Steiner H. Stimulus-Dependent Expression of Immediate-Early Genes in Rat Somatosensory Cortex. J Comp Neurol 1997;380:145–153.

[91] Masri S, Sassone-Corsi P. The circadian clock: a framework linking metabolism, epigenetics and neuronal function. Nature Rev Neurosci 2013;14: 69-75.

[92] Hayakawa K, Hirosawa M, Tabei Y, Arai D, Tanaka S, Murakami N, Yagi S, Shiota K. Epigenetic switching by the metabolism-sensing factors in the generation of orexin neurons from mouse embryonic stem cells. J Biol Chem 2013;288(24):17099-110.

[93] Duarte AI, Moreira PI, Oliveira CR. Insulin in Central Nervous System: More than Just a Peripheral Hormone. J Aging Res 2012, Article ID 384017. doi: 10.1155/2012/384017.

[94] Stone WS, Seidman LJ. Toward a Model of Memory Enhancement in Schizophrenia: Glucose Administration and Hippocampal Function. Schizophr Bull 2008; 34 (1): 93–108.

[95] Choi S-W, Friso S. Epigenetics: A New Bridge between Nutrition and Health. Adv Nutr 2010; 1: 8–16.

[96] Benton D, Parker PY. Breakfast, blood glucose, and cognition. Am J Clin Nutr 1998;67(suppl):772S–8S.

[97] Li T, Chanda D, Zhang Y, Choi HS, Chiang JY. Glucose stimulates cholesterol 7 β-hydroxylase gene transcription in human hepatocytes. J Lipid Res 2010. 51: 832–842.

[98] Kaelin Jr. WG, McKnight SL. Influence of Metabolism on Epigenetics and Disease. Cell 2013;153: 56-69.

[99] Lu C, Thompson CB. Metabolic regulation of epigenetics. Cell Metab 2012; 16(1): 9–17.

[100] Bouchard L, Thibault S, Guay S-P, Santure M, Monpetit A, St-Pierre J, Perron P, Brisson D. Leptin Gene Epigenetic Adaptation to Impaired Glucose Metabolism During Pregnancy. Diabetes Care 2010;33:2436–2441.

[101] Jufvas Ås, Sjödin S, Lundqvist K, Amin R, Vener AV, Strålfors P. Global differences in specific histone H3 methylation are associated with overweight and type 2 diabetes. Clin Epigen 2013, 5:15.

[102] Jayaraman S. Epigenetic Mechanisms of Metabolic Memory in Diabetes. Circ Res 2012;110:1039-1041.

[103] Schiöth HB, Craft S, Brooks SJ, Frey II WH, Benedict C. Brain Insulin Signaling and Alzheimer's Disease: Current Evidence and Future Directions. Mol Neurobiol 2012; 46:4–10.

[104] de la Monte SM. Insulin resistance and Alzheimer's disease. BMB reports 2009;42(8): 475-481.

[105] Arnáiz E, Jelic V, Almkvist O, Wahlund L-O, Winblad B, Valind S, Nordberg A. Impaired cerebral glucose metabolism and cognitive functioning predict deterioration in mild cognitive impairment. Neuroreport 2001; 12 (4):851-855.

[106] Freiherr J, Hallschmid M, Frey WH 2nd, Brünner YF, Chapman CD, Hölscher C, Craft S, De Felice FG, Benedict C. Intranasal Insulin as a Treatment for Alzheimer's Disease: A Review of Basic Research and Clinical Evidence. CNS Drugs 2013; 27:505–514.

[107] Schapiro MB, Ball MJ, Grady CL, Haxby JV, Kaye JA, Rapoport SI. Dementia in Down's syndrome: cerebral glucose utilization, neuropsychological assessment, and neuropathology. Neurology 1988;38(6):938-42.

[108] Pietrini P, Dani A, Furey ML, Alexander GE, Freo U, Grady CL, Mentis MJ, Mangot D, Simon EW, Horwitz B, Haxby JV, Schapiro MB. Low glucose metabolism during brain stimulation in older Down's syndrome subjects at risk for Alzheimer's disease prior to dementia. Am J Psychiatry 1997;154(8):1063-9.

[109] Roffman JL, Nitenson AZ, Agam Y, Isom M, Friedman JS, Dyckman KA, Brohawn DG, Smoller JW, Goff DC, Manoach DS. A hypomethylating variant of MTHFR, 677C>T, blunts the neural response to errors in patients with schizophrenia and healthy individuals. PLoS One. 2011;6(9):e25253. doi: 10.1371/journal.pone.0025253.

[110] Jokeit H, Seitz RJ, Markowitsch HJ, Neumann N, Witte OW, Ebner A. Prefrontal asymmetric interictal glucose hypometabolism and cognitive impairment in patients with temporal lobe epilepsy. BRAIN 1997; 120: 2283–2294.

[111] Siegel BV Jr, Buchsbaum MS, Bunney WE Jr, Gottschalk LA, Haier RJ, Lohr JB, Lottenberg S, Najafi A, Nuechterlein KH, Potkin SG, et al. Cortical-striatal-thalamic circuits and brain glucose metabolic activity in 70 unmedicated male schizophrenic patients. Am J Psychiatry 1993;150(9):1325-36.

[112] Buchsbaum MS, Haier RJ, Potkin SG, Nuechterlein K, Bracha HS, Katz M, et al. Frontostriatal disorder of cerebral metabolism in never-medicated schizophrenics. Arch Gen Psychiatry 1992;49(12):935-42.

[113] Peppard RF, Martin WRW, Clark CM, Carr GD, McGeer PL, Calne DB. Cortical glucose metabolism in parkinson's and alzheimer's disease. J Neurosci Res 1990; 27 (4): 561–568.

[114] Shkil'nyuk GG, Il'ves AG, Kataeva GV, Prakhova LN, Reznikova TN, Seliverstova NA, Stolyarov ID. The Role of Changes in Glucose Metabolism in the Brain in the Formation of Cognitive Impairments in Patients with Remitting and Secondary-Progressive Multiple Sclerosis. Neurosci Behav Physiol 2013; 43 (5):565-570.

[115] Holroyd CB, Praamstra P, Plat E, Coles MGH. Spared error-related potentials in mild to moderate Parkinson's disease. Neuropsychologia. 2002; 40: 2116–2124.

[116] Holroyd CB, Yeung N. Alcohol and error processing. Trends Neurosci 2003; 26: 402-404.

[117] Hester R, Foxe JJ, Molholm S, Shpaner M, Garavan H. Neural mechanisms involved in error processing: a comparison of errors made with and without awareness. NeuroImage. 2005; 27: 602–608.

[118] Yazan Alderazi, Francesca Brett. Alcohol and the nervous system. Curr Diagn Pathol 2007; 13: 203–209.

Section 3

Adipokines, TRH and Cells

Chapter 6

Adipokines Involved in Macrophage Recruitment

Dayea Kim, Jong Hyuk Yoon, Jaeyoon Kim and
Sung Ho Ryu

Additional information is available at the end of the chapter

http://dx.doi.org/10.5772/57558

1. Introduction

Recent studies have reported adipose tissue as a crucial site for the generation of inflammatory responses and mediators in metabolic syndrome. In addition to the intrinsic properties of adipocytes in energy storage and metabolic homeostasis, adipose tissue serves as a key area for the interaction of adipocytes with other factors of the immune system.

An important feature of inflammation is recruitment of immune cells such as neutrophils, eosinophils, and macrophages. Macrophage infiltration of adipose tissue in obese conditions has been studied in both mice and humans. It has been suggested that expanding adipocytes or neighboring pre-adipocytes could start to produce chemotactic signals inducing to macrophage recruitment, and this event is linked to systemic inflammation and insulin resistance.

In this chapter, we describe several chemotactic factors that have been implicated in the recruitment of inflammatory monocytes and macrophages into adipose tissue.

2. Body

2.1. Adipose tissue inflammation

2.1.1. Adipose tissue as a site of inflammation: expansion of adipose tissue induces an inflammatory response that contributes to metabolic disorders

2.1.1.1. Composition and function of adipose tissue

Adipose tissue is connective tissue composed primarily of adipocytes. The highest percentage of cells within adipose tissue is adipocytes; other cell types present in adipose tissue are collectively termed the stromal vascular fraction (SVF), which includes pre-adipocytes, adipose tissue macrophages, fibroblasts, and endothelial cells. Adipose tissue primarily plays a role in the storage of energy in the form of lipids when nutrients are in excess or in the regulation of homeostasis of non-shivering thermogenesis. Adipose tissue regulates whole body energy homeostasis by responding rapidly and dynamically to changes in nutrient deprivation and excess through regulation of adipocyte size and number [1, 2]. In this reaction, free fatty acids (FFAs) are released from lipoproteins by lipoprotein lipase (LPL) and enter the adipocyte, where they are reassembled into triglycerides by esterification onto glycerol. Adipose tissue also provides feedback for hunger and diet to the brain under normal conditions through secretion of hormones [3].

2.1.1.2. Adipose tissue mediates obesity-induced inflammation

Obesity negatively affects the functioning of peripheral tissues, including adipose tissue, skeletal muscle, the pancreas, liver, heart, joints, and central nervous system (CNS) [4]. The fundamental characteristic of obesity is chronic imbalance between caloric intake and energy expenditure, resulting in the storage of excess nutrients in white adipose tissue (WAT) [5]. WAT was traditionally considered a long-term energy storage organ, but it is now known that it has a key role in the systemic regulation of metabolism. The metabolic function is largely mediated by the ability of WAT to secrete numerous proteins [6, 7]. The cytokines secreted by adipose tissue are called adipokines. In the obese state, the secretory status of adipose tissue is modified by changes in the cellular composition, including diverse alterations in the number, phenotype, and localization of immune, vascular, and structural cells [6]. Adipose tissue in obese human patients and in animal models of obesity are infiltrated by a large number of macrophages, and this recruitment is linked to systemic inflammation and insulin resistance [8, 9]. The secretion of most adipokines is upregulated in the obese state, and these proteins primarily include proinflammatory cytokines such as monocyte chemotactic protein-1 (MCP-1), TNF-α, and interleukin (IL)-6, which function to promote the development of a chronic and systemic inflammatory state and contribute to metabolic dysfunction [6, 10, 11]. Therefore, adipose tissue-mediated inflammation is a considered to be a pathophysiological condition (Figure 1).

Increased levels of the cytokine TNF-α in adipose tissue of obese mice were the first discovered link between inflammation and obesity [12]. This discovery was soon followed by many studies describing changes in the levels of inflammatory molecules between obese and lean states in animals as well as humans. It is now known that, in addition to TNF-α, an array of inflammatory cytokines including IL-6, IL-1β, MCP-1, and others are increased in obese tissues [13, 14].

2.1.2. Obesity-mediated macrophage recruitment into adipose tissue and metabolic disease

It is generally accepted that obesity causes adipocytes to secrete chemokines such as MCP-1 and leukotriene B4 (LTB4), which provide a chemotactic gradient that recruits monocytes into adipose tissue, where they become adipose tissue macrophages (ATMs) (Figure 2). Once proinflammatory ATMs migrate into adipose tissue, they also secrete their own cytokines,

http://dx.doi.org/10.5772/57558

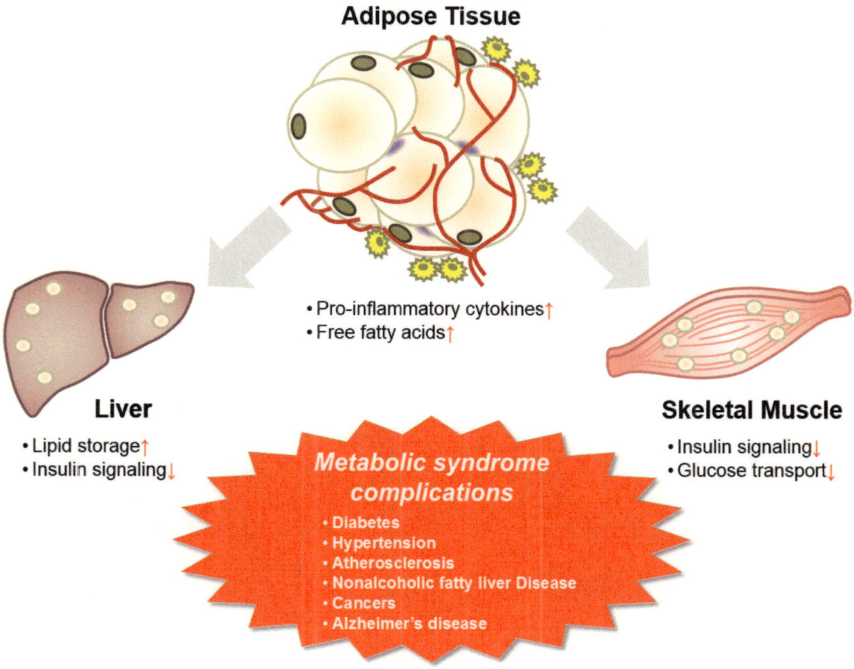

Figure 1. Adipose tissue affects peripheral metabolic tissues and induces diverse metabolic syndrome complications

recruit additional macrophages, and ultimately set up an amplified inflammatory process [15]. Specifically, ATMs together with hypertrophic adipocytes, pre-adipocytes, and other immune cells produce an array of chemokines, proinflammatory cytokines, and metabolites that induce endothelial activation during obesity. This reaction causes endothelial cells to produce various cellular adhesion molecules such as ICAMs, selectins, vascular cell adhesion molecules, and PECAM-1. Through a rolling and adhesion step, monocytes slow down and finally bind to endothelial adhesion proteins via selectin ligands and integrins. After a series of events including actin-dependent spreading, polarization, the monocytes undergo integrin-dependent lateral migration on the luminal surface of the endothelium. Then, the monocytes migrate across the endothelium, either through para-or transcellular routes [16]. After entering adipose tissue, macrophages undergo differentiation towards M1-or M2-like macrophages (See Section 2.2) [17]. Differentiation processes can occur according to their initial circulating phenotype and/or in response to local micro-environmental stimuli. However, repolarization of M1 macrophages into M2 macrophages and conversely, proliferation of macrophages within the adipose tissue still remain unclear [17].

The recruitment of macrophages into adipose tissue is the initial and important event in obesity-induced inflammation and metabolic disease [15]. Activation of tissue macrophages, as the outcome, triggers the secretion of proinflammatory cytokines, which can induce insulin resistance in various pathways. Genetic studies using knockout (KO) and transgenic techniques to disable macrophage-mediated inflammatory pathways also support this pathway [15].

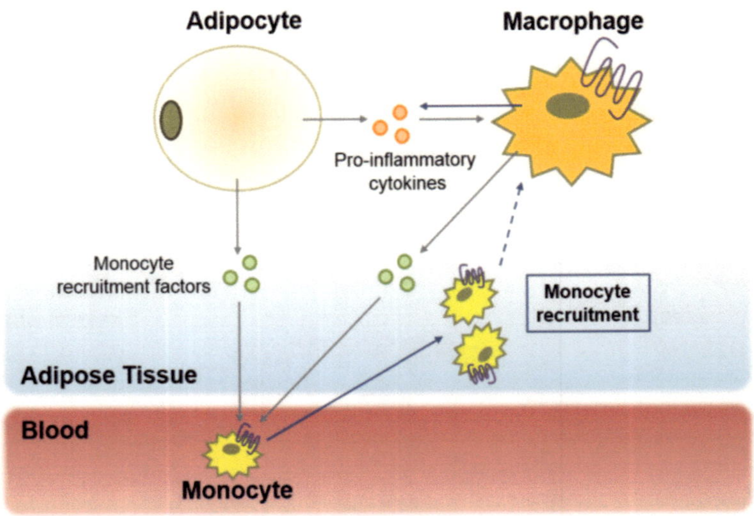

Figure 2. Adipokines induce obesity-mediated immune cell recruitment into adipose tissue

2.2. Adipose tissue macrophages: types and functions in metabolic disease

2.2.1. Origin and function of ATM

Pre-adipocytes have been shown to convert to macrophages [18], but most ATMs migrate from blood monocytes during obesity. Bone-marrow transplantation experiments using transgenic mice with antigenically distinct forms of the CD45 protein, a leukocyte marker, showed that 85% of ATMs after 6 weeks of a high fat diet (HFD) were from donor cells, which indicates that blood circulating monocytes migrated into adipose tissue while receiving the HFD [9]. Therefore, there are likely some signals that attract blood monocytes to adipose tissue (see Section 2.3). Since ATMs are the primary source for proinflammatory cytokines in adipose tissue, it was hypothesized that ATMs might be the critical player for systemic insulin resistance. Several studies have supported this hypothesis in *in vivo* models. For example, myeloid-specific IKKβ KO mice showed improved insulin sensitivity with the HFD [19], and mice with JNK1 and 2 deficiencies in macrophages were obese but were still insulin sensitive with fewer macrophages and lower proinflammatory cytokine expression in adipose tissues [20]. These studies suggested that changes in macrophage activation might affect whole body insulin sensitivity.

2.2.2. General aspects of macrophage activation

Macrophages are a heterogeneous cell population exhibiting a wide spectrum of phenotypes due to cellular differentiation, wide spread tissue distribution, and responsiveness to many endogenous and exogenous stimuli. Macrophage activation has been defined across 2 separate polarization states, M1 and M2 [21]. M1 macrophages are referred to as classical activated macrophages where activation is dependent on products of specifically activated T helper 1 (T_H1)-type lymphocytes and natural killer cells. Similar to interferon-gamma (IFN-γ) [22] and IL-12, IL-18 is presented by antigen presenting cells (APCs). M1 macrophages secrete high levels of proinflammatory cytokines (TNF-α, IL-6, IL-12) and generate reactive oxygen species (ROS) through the actions of inducible nitric oxide synthase (NOS2). M2 macrophages are activated by IL-4 and IL-13, cytokines produced generally in a T_H-2-type response, which is referred to as alternative activation. This type of activation is believed to be involved in allergic, cellular, and humoral responses to parasitic and extracellular pathogens. M2 macrophages secrete low levels of proinflammatory cytokines and high level of anti-inflammatory cytokines [21]. Three different subsets of M2 macrophages have been identified, including M2a, M2b, and M2c. IL-4 and IL-13 lead to M2a macrophages, immune complexes in combination with IL-1b or lipopolysaccharide (LPS) drive the M2b subtype, whereas IL-10, TGF-β, or glucocorticoids induce M2c macrophages [23]. In alternative activation, IL-4 and IL-13 upregulate expression of the mannose receptor and MHC class II molecules, which stimulate endocytosis and antigen, while intracellular enzymes such as arginase are implicated in cell recruitment and granuloma formation.

2.2.3. Activation of adipose tissue macrophages (ATMs)

Originally, ATMs were suggested to have roles in the production of proinflammatory cytokines [8, 9]; therefore, it seems plausible that most ATMs are M1 macrophages in obesity. In initial pioneering studies regarding ATMs, ATM content was determined by F4/80 or CD11b antibodies, which are common macrophage markers that cannot differentiate between M1 and M2 macrophages. Subsequent studies have shown that ATMs are operationally defined across M1 to M2 polarization states. Using flow cytometry, it was shown that ATM from lean mice showed the M2 macrophage phenotype, but ATMs that accumulated following a HFD exhibited the proinflammatory M1 phenotype. Based on these data, it was suggested that ATMs underwent a phenotypic switch from the M2 polarization state to a more M1 polarization state [24]. In line with ATM polarization, ATMs with M1-like activation were characterized by F4/80$^+$/CD11b$^+$/CD11c$^+$surface markers, whereas F4/80$^+$/CD11b$^+$/CD11c$^-$cells were present following M2-like activation [24, 25]. Since F4/80 and CD11c were primarily considered as surface markers for macrophages and dendritic cells, respectively, these ATMs with triple positive surface markers are unusual in that they have both macrophage and dendritic cell features [25]. These data are supported by the fact that CD11c$^+$cells have a deleterious effect on insulin resistance; it was shown that selective depletion of CD11c$^+$cells reversed insulin resistance with a HFD [26]. A recent article showed the temporal dynamics of macrophage activation where it was shown that M2 ATM polarization was enhanced in the early phase of obesity (both in the *ob*/*ob* model and the diet-induced obesity (DIO) model), and M1 polarization was subsequently gradually enhanced [27]. These data indicate that there are temporal and spatio differences between M1 and M2 macrophages during obesity. While M2 macrophages (resident macrophages) were localized to interstitial spaces between adipocytes in lean mice, M1 ATMs surrounded dead adipocytes with DIO, thus forming crown-like structures

(CLSs) [28]. However, the activation status of ATMs does not seem to be static. Whereas HFD-induced insulin resistance followed by a normal chow diet could reverse body insulin sensitivity, mice still contained a similar level of $CD11c^+$ATMs in adipose tissue, but these macrophages no longer exhibited inflammatory pathway markers [29]. Furthermore, a class of macrophages that express a marker for both M1 and M2 (i.e., $CD11c^+$, $CD209a^+$) was identified in obese adipose tissues. These macrophages were likely transformed from M2 to M1 macrophages through lipid accumulation [27]. Therefore, there might be some mechanism to regulate activation of ATMs in adipose tissue along with obesity development.

2.2.4. Regulation of ATM polarization

Classical activation of macrophages (M1) is induced by Toll-like receptor (TLR) ligands and IFN-γ, while alternative activation of macrophages (M2) is induced by IL-4/IL-13 (M2a), immune complexes (M2b), or anti-inflammatory cytokines IL-10 or TGF-β (M2c) to mediate Th1/Th2 immune responses [30]. In the classical activation of macrophages, adipose tissue secretes FFAs, which can activate TLR4 [31] by lipolysis and IFN-γ. On the other hand, it was shown that adipocytes secrete Th2 cytokines such as IL-4 and IL-13, which is important for alternative macrophage activation [32]. Adiponectin is also reported to induce M2 polarization, which was shown using adiponectin KO mice and adenoviral delivery of adiponectin [33].

In terms of intracellular signaling in adipose tissue macrophages, transcription factors and related machinery that regulate ATM polarization have been studied. Peroxisome proliferator–activated receptor gamma (PPARγ) is one of most striking regulators because it is known as a master regulator of adipogenesis. However, PPARγ was expressed at relatively high levels in monocytes and macrophages [34], and it was reported that PPARγ activation reduced proinflammatory cytokines in monocytes/macrophages [35, 36]. When PPARγ was knocked out in macrophages, bone marrow-derived macrophages showed impaired alternative macrophage activation, and these mice were obese, with an insulin resistant and glucose intolerant phenotype following HFD feeding [37]. PPARδ, another PPAR family member, is also important for ATM polarization. Myeloid-specific KO of PPARδ resulted in enhanced adipose tissue inflammation and insulin resistance, which is consistent with the M1 polarization phenotype [32]. PGC-1β, a co-activator of the PPAR family, is also clearly involved in alternative macrophage activation by cooperating with STAT6, which is a critical signal mediated by Th2 cytokines [38]. In addition, Krüppel-like factor 4 (KLF4), which belongs to the zinc finger class of DNA-binding transcriptional regulators, was suggested to be a master regulator of macrophage polarization during obesity. KLF4 expression was markedly reduced in obese adipose tissue, and KLF4 deficiency exhibited an enhanced inflammatory response. In particular, myeloid specific KO of KLF4 led to obesity, insulin resistance, and impaired glucose tolerance [39]. Interferon regulatory factor 4 (IRF4) is also known to be involved in ATM polarization. Macrophage-specific IRF4 KO mice exhibited significant insulin resistance and adipose tissue inflammation with a HFD [40].

http://dx.doi.org/10.5772/57558

2.3. Adipose tissue-derived chemotactic factors and macrophage recruitment in metabolic diseases

Human studies and mouse models have both been used to identify the chemokines and associated receptors that are elevated in obese adipose tissue [41] and those that contribute to monocyte recruitment [17].

2.3.1. MCP-1 and CCR2

MCP-1 (CCL2) is produced mostly by macrophages and endothelial cells and is a potent chemotactic factor for monocytes [42-44]. The level of MCP-1 in both WAT and plasma was increased in obese mice [45], suggesting that MCP-1 might be an adipokine whose expression is increased in obesity [46].

Binding of MCP-1 to its receptor CCR2 is considered crucial in obesity-induced insulin resistance. Several groups have demonstrated that mice with targeted deletions in the genes for *Mcp-1* and its receptor *Ccr2* have decreased ATM content, decreased inflammation in WAT, and protection against obesity-induced insulin resistance [46, 47]. On the contrary to this, mice overexpressing MCP-1 in adipose tissue had increased ATM and insulin resistance [46, 48]. Therefore, the MCP-1-CCR2 axis is important to promote ATM recruitment and insulin resistance in mice. Recent studies; however, have shown conflicting results and indicate a greater complexity than suggested by previous reports. In studies done by several groups, results showed that loss of MCP-1 did not attenuate obesity-associated macrophage recruitment to WAT or improve metabolic function, suggesting that MCP-1 is not pivotal for obesity-induced macrophage recruitment and systemic insulin resistance [49, 50]. Furthermore, although *Ccr2*$^{-/-}$mice fed a HFD had fewer macrophages in WAT compared with wild type (WT) mice [47], CCR2 deficiency did not normalize ATM content and insulin resistance to the levels in lean mice, indicating that ATM recruitment and insulin resistance are also regulated by MCP-1-CCR2 independent signals. The intricacy and redundancy of chemokine signaling may account for these conflicting results.

2.3.2. CCL3, CCL5, CCR1, and CCR5

Macrophage inflammatory protein-1 (MIP-1/CCL3) is a CC chemokine with upregulated expression in obese WAT of humans and mice. CCL3 transcript and protein are remarkably elevated in WAT of *ob*/*ob*, *db*/*db*, and DIO mice [8, 51]. In obese humans, the expression of CCL3 and its receptors CCR1 and CCR5 were increased in omental and subcutaneous WAT compared with normal weight individuals [41]. Moreover, expression of CCL3 and CCR1 in WAT was positively correlated with fasting blood insulin levels in humans [41, 52, 53]. Although many reports have shown a functional role of CCL3 in obesity, the consequences of this have not been established [54].

Keophiphath et al. identified CCL5 as the most upregulated gene in human pre-adipocytes provided with macrophage-secreted factors [55]. Although its role and its target receptors in human WAT are unknown, this chemokine is involved in blood monocyte recruitment to inflammatory sites by binding to the G-protein-coupled receptors CCR1, CCR3, and CCR5.

CCL5 production in fibroblasts, platelets, and monocytes/macrophages is a known feature of inflammatory disorders [56]. In atherosclerosis, CCL5, via CCR1 and CCR5, contributes to transmigration of monocytes and T cells in atherogenic lesions [57].

Kitade et al. revealed that CCR5 plays a crucial role in the regulation of adipose tissue inflammation in obesity and the development of insulin resistance [58]. Expression of CCR5 and its ligands is highly increased in WAT of both *ob*/*ob* and DIO mice. FACS analysis clearly demonstrated that $CCR5^{+}$macrophages accumulate in WAT of obese mice. The loss of CCR5 improved obesity-induced insulin resistance in mice. Both *Ccr5*$^{-/-}$mice fed a HFD and mice deficient in *Ccr5* bone marrow-derived cells showed ameliorated insulin sensitivity and protection from obesity-induced insulin resistance via reduction of ATM accumulation.

2.3.3. LTB4 and BLT-1

LTB4 is a kind of proinflammatory lipid mediator generated from arachidonic acid [59, 60]. LTB4 is rapidly produced by activated leukocytes, it promotes leukocyte chemotaxis, and regulates proinflammatory cytokines [59, 61]. The biological actions of LTB4 are mediated by an interaction with a G protein-coupled receptor termed BLT-1 [61]. Although the LTB4/BLT-1 axis plays a critical role in host defense during acute infection, chronic activation of this pathway provides continuous inflammation, which is feature of inflammatory pathologies such as atherosclerosis and arthritis [62-67]. Moreover, LTB4 levels increased in adipose tissue of both mice and rats consuming a HFD [67-69]. Spite et al. reported that deficiency of BLT-1 protects against the progression of insulin resistance in DIO by regulating ATM accumulation and inflammation in peripheral tissues [70].

2.3.4. Fractalkine (CX3CL1) and CX3CR1

CX3CL1, a chemokine that binds to a single known receptor (CX3CR1), is involved in the recruitment and adhesion of both monocytes and T cells in atherosclerosis and rheumatologic disorders [71]. CX3CR1 is a G-protein-coupled receptor expressed in many leukocyte subtypes [72, 73] and promotes leukocyte activation and survival [74]. To develop macrophage-rich atherosclerotic lesions, CX3CR1 is required for monocyte recruitment. [75, 76]. Digby et al. suggested that adipocytes also expressed CX3CL1 and that CX3CR1 signaling in macrophages was inhibited by PPARγ agonists [77]. Moreover, modulation of the CX3CL1/CX3CR1 system can regulate chronic inflammatory diseases, including atherosclerosis, independent of CCL2/CCR2 [78], which indicates that this also occur in adipose tissue inflammation and its related complications. Recently, Shah et al. found that CX3CL1 is one of markedly upregulated genes in human adipose tissue through *in vivo* inflammation by using a microarray of adipose tissue mRNA during experimental endotoxemia [79, 80].

2.3.5. CXCL14

CXCL14 (originally designated as BRAK, BMAC, or Mip-2g) is expressed in WAT, brown adipose tissue (BAT), and skeletal muscle, which indicates that it may have a role in adipogenesis, myogenesis, and metabolic complications. CXCL14, as a chemoattractant, is required for activated tissue macrophages and dendritic cells [81-87]. Nara et al. generated *Cxcl14* deficient mice and described that CXCL14 is involved in the obesity-induced infiltration of macrophages into WAT, serum adipokine levels, hepatic steatosis, and attenuation of insulin signaling in skeletal muscle; thereby, contributing to systemic insulin resistance in DIO mice [88].

2.3.6. Osteopontin

Osteopontin (OPN) is a secreted matrix glycoprotein and proinflammatory cytokine that has previously been reported as a major element of cell-mediated immunity [89]. Many studies have provided evidence that OPN is secreted by macrophages at sites of inflammation where it mediates monocyte adhesion [90], migration [91], differentiation [92], and phagocytosis [93]. OPN play a role in the development of atherosclerosis. OPN induces chemotaxis of monocytes and elevates cellular migration through a direct interaction with its receptors [94, 95]. Nomiyama et al. demonstrated that OPN secretion is upregulated during obesity and greatly expressed in ATMs of DIO mice, characterizing OPN as an adipokine. OPN deficiency attenuated ATM accumulation, adipose tissue inflammation and improved whole body insulin resistance [96].

2.3.7. Apoptosis inhibitor of macrophage (AIM/CD5L)

AIM [97] is incorporated into adipocytes via CD36-associated endocytosis, and it mediated lipolysis by suppressing the activity of fatty acid synthase (FAS) [98]. AIM is a member of the scavenger receptor cysteine-rich superfamily and was initially characterized as an apoptosis inhibitor that supports the survival of macrophages against apoptosis-inducing stimuli [97]. AIM is a direct target for regulation by nuclear receptor liver X receptor/retinoid X receptor (LXR/RXR) heterodimers [99, 100], and it is exclusively produced by tissue macrophages. As a secreted molecule, AIM is found in both human and mouse blood [97, 100-103] and increases in blood with the progression of obesity in DIO mice [98]. AIM-associated lipolysis is responsible for the obesity-induced recruitment of ATMs. Kurokawa et al. demonstrated the role of AIM in the initiation of adipose tissue inflammation that links obesity and insulin resistance [104]. Firstly, AIM-induced lipolysis is required for macrophage recruitment into obese adipose tissues. Increased blood AIM levels induce dynamic lipolysis in obese adipose tissues, augmenting local extracellular fatty acid concentrations to a level sufficient for the stimulation of TLR4, which promotes chemokine production by adipocytes and macrophage infiltration. Secondly, an increase in blood AIM is required as well as adipocyte hypertrophy for the initiation of macrophage recruitment. In *AIM* deficient mice, although the level of AIM-independent lipolysis escalated in line with adipocyte hypertrophy [98], it may not reach a level sufficient for macrophage infiltration. Thirdly, crosstalk between adipocytes and macrophages within adipose tissue establishes a vicious circle that accelerates inflammation; saturated fatty acids brought about by lipolysis activated TLR4 to induce TNFα, which in turn activated the TNFα receptor to produce inflammatory cytokines [105]. This response induces a further progression of inflammation, lipolysis, and macrophage recruitment.

2.3.8. Macrophage migration inhibitory factor (MIF)

MIF is a multifunctional proinflammatory cytokine which is responsible for inflammatory processes. The primary source and target of MIF have been identified as macrophages [106]. MIF is rapidly released in response to inflammatory stimuli such as lipopolysaccharide, TNF-α, and IFN-γ. MIF can have both paracrine and autocrine effects [106-108]. MIF elevates adipose tissue inflammation through amplification of migration, recruitment, and activation of leukocytes at the site of inflammation through upregulation of adhesion molecules such as ICAM-1 and MCP-1 [109-111]. MIF can utilize its chemotactic properties via CXCR2 and CXCR4 in macrophages and T cells, respectively [111]. The interaction of MIF with CXCR4 on the surface of fibroblasts and T cells induced CXCL8 secretion [112]. Interestingly, the alternative MIF receptor CD74, which is traditionally involved in the activation of the mitogen-activated protein kinases pathway, has recently been demonstrated to also mediate macrophage chemotactic responses [113, 114]. Although these roles in macrophage recruitment have been demonstrated, a recent study showed MIF-/-mice did not exhibit significant changes in ATM content compared to WT mice when fed a HFD [115].

3. Conclusion

Adipose tissue inflammation and macrophage infiltration are well-established features of obesity. ATMs are separated into at least two groups: M1 and M2. In obesity, more than 90% of recruited monocytes become M1 macrophages that can secrete proinflammatory cytokines resulting in adipose tissue inflammation and insulin resistance. Many studies have identified adipokines that can recruit monocytes into adipose tissue in obesity. Consequently, adipose tissue-derived chemokines may be promising therapeutic targets for insulin resistance and metabolic diseases. Although modulation of a single chemokine can affect the chemotaxis of monocytes when they are studied individually, it is likely that chemokines have overlapping functions in the more complex *in vivo* environment. Moreover, the complicated process of monocyte recruitment and subsequent differentiation into M1 or M2 macrophages in obese adipose tissue appears to be substantially different in mouse and human obesity, which emphasizes the need for investigations in humans. Therefore, whether macrophage depletion stands for an appropriate tool to ameliorate adipose tissue homeostasis and restore insulin resistance in obesity remains an open question.

Acknowledgements

This work was supported by the National Research Foundation of Korea(NRF) grant funded by the Korea government(MEST) (No. 2013R1A2A1A03010110 and No.2010-0028684).

http://dx.doi.org/10.5772/57558

Author details

Dayea Kim[1], Jong Hyuk Yoon[1], Jaeyoon Kim[2] and Sung Ho Ryu[1*]

*Address all correspondence to: sungho@postech.ac.kr

1 Department of Life Sciences, Pohang University of Science and Technology (POSTECH), Pohang, Gyeongbuk, Republic of Korea

2 The Rolf Luft Research Center for Diabetes and Endocrinology, Karolinska Institutet, Stockholm, Sweden

References

[1] Sun K, Kusminski CM, Scherer PE. Adipose tissue remodeling and obesity. The Journal of clinical investigation. 2011 Jun;121(6):2094-101. PubMed PMID: 21633177. Pubmed Central PMCID: 3104761.

[2] Aarsland A, Chinkes D, Wolfe RR. Hepatic and whole-body fat synthesis in humans during carbohydrate overfeeding. The American journal of clinical nutrition. 1997 Jun;65(6):1774-82. PubMed PMID: 9174472.

[3] Henry BA, Clarke IJ. Adipose tissue hormones and the regulation of food intake. Journal of neuroendocrinology. 2008 Jun;20(6):842-9. PubMed PMID: 18601708.

[4] Ferrante AW, Jr. Obesity-induced inflammation: a metabolic dialogue in the language of inflammation. Journal of internal medicine. 2007 Oct;262(4):408-14. PubMed PMID: 17875176.

[5] Odegaard JI, Chawla A. Pleiotropic actions of insulin resistance and inflammation in metabolic homeostasis. Science. 2013 Jan 11;339(6116):172-7. PubMed PMID: 23307735. Pubmed Central PMCID: 3725457.

[6] Ouchi N, Parker JL, Lugus JJ, Walsh K. Adipokines in inflammation and metabolic disease. Nature reviews Immunology. 2011 Feb;11(2):85-97. PubMed PMID: 21252989. Pubmed Central PMCID: 3518031.

[7] Wynn TA, Chawla A, Pollard JW. Macrophage biology in development, homeostasis and disease. Nature. 2013 Apr 25;496(7446):445-55. PubMed PMID: 23619691. Pubmed Central PMCID: 3725458.

[8] Xu H, Barnes GT, Yang Q, Tan G, Yang D, Chou CJ, et al. Chronic inflammation in fat plays a crucial role in the development of obesity-related insulin resistance. The Journal of clinical investigation. 2003 Dec;112(12):1821-30. PubMed PMID: 14679177. Pubmed Central PMCID: 296998.

[9] Weisberg SP, McCann D, Desai M, Rosenbaum M, Leibel RL, Ferrante AW, Jr. Obesity is associated with macrophage accumulation in adipose tissue. The Journal of clinical investigation. 2003 Dec;112(12):1796-808. PubMed PMID: 14679176. Pubmed Central PMCID: 296995.

[10] Yoon JH, Kim J, Song P, Lee TG, Suh PG, Ryu SH. Secretomics for skeletal muscle cells: a discovery of novel regulators? Advances in biological regulation. 2012 May; 52(2):340-50. PubMed PMID: 22781747.

[11] Kershaw EE, Flier JS. Adipose tissue as an endocrine organ. The Journal of clinical endocrinology and metabolism. 2004 Jun;89(6):2548-56. PubMed PMID: 15181022.

[12] Hotamisligil GS, Arner P, Caro JF, Atkinson RL, Spiegelman BM. Increased adipose tissue expression of tumor necrosis factor-alpha in human obesity and insulin resistance. The Journal of clinical investigation. 1995 May;95(5):2409-15. PubMed PMID: 7738205. Pubmed Central PMCID: 295872.

[13] Shoelson SE, Lee J, Goldfine AB. Inflammation and insulin resistance. The Journal of clinical investigation. 2006 Jul;116(7):1793-801. PubMed PMID: 16823477. Pubmed Central PMCID: 1483173.

[14] Berg AH, Scherer PE. Adipose tissue, inflammation, and cardiovascular disease. Circulation research. 2005 May 13;96(9):939-49. PubMed PMID: 15890981.

[15] Osborn O, Olefsky JM. The cellular and signaling networks linking the immune system and metabolism in disease. Nature medicine. 2012 Mar;18(3):363-74. PubMed PMID: 22395709.

[16] Kamei M, Carman CV. New observations on the trafficking and diapedesis of monocytes. Current opinion in hematology. 2010 Jan;17(1):43-52. PubMed PMID: 19996887.

[17] Dalmas E, Clement K, Guerre-Millo M. Defining macrophage phenotype and function in adipose tissue. Trends in immunology. 2011 Jul;32(7):307-14. PubMed PMID: 21616718. Epub 2011/05/28. eng.

[18] Charriere G, Cousin B, Arnaud E, Andre M, Bacou F, Penicaud L, et al. Preadipocyte conversion to macrophage. Evidence of plasticity. The Journal of biological chemistry. 2003 Mar 14;278(11):9850-5. PubMed PMID: 12519759.

[19] Arkan MC, Hevener AL, Greten FR, Maeda S, Li ZW, Long JM, et al. IKK-beta links inflammation to obesity-induced insulin resistance. Nature medicine. 2005 Feb;11(2): 191-8. PubMed PMID: 15685170.

[20] Han MS, Jung DY, Morel C, Lakhani SA, Kim JK, Flavell RA, et al. JNK expression by macrophages promotes obesity-induced insulin resistance and inflammation. Science. 2013 Jan 11;339(6116):218-22. PubMed PMID: 23223452.

[21] Gordon S. Alternative activation of macrophages. Nature reviews Immunology. 2003 Jan;3(1):23-35. PubMed PMID: 12511873.

[22] Dalton DK, Pitts-Meek S, Keshav S, Figari IS, Bradley A, Stewart TA. Multiple defects of immune cell function in mice with disrupted interferon-gamma genes. Science. 1993 Mar 19;259(5102):1739-42. PubMed PMID: 8456300.

[23] Chinetti-Gbaguidi G, Staels B. Macrophage polarization in metabolic disorders: functions and regulation. Current opinion in lipidology. 2011 Oct;22(5):365-72. PubMed PMID: 21825981. Pubmed Central PMCID: 3565956.

[24] Lumeng CN, Bodzin JL, Saltiel AR. Obesity induces a phenotypic switch in adipose tissue macrophage polarization. The Journal of clinical investigation. 2007 Jan;117(1): 175-84. PubMed PMID: 17200717. Pubmed Central PMCID: 1716210.

[25] Nguyen MT, Favelyukis S, Nguyen AK, Reichart D, Scott PA, Jenn A, et al. A subpopulation of macrophages infiltrates hypertrophic adipose tissue and is activated by free fatty acids via Toll-like receptors 2 and 4 and JNK-dependent pathways. The Journal of biological chemistry. 2007 Nov 30;282(48):35279-92. PubMed PMID: 17916553.

[26] Patsouris D, Li PP, Thapar D, Chapman J, Olefsky JM, Neels JG. Ablation of CD11c-positive cells normalizes insulin sensitivity in obese insulin resistant animals. Cell metabolism. 2008 Oct;8(4):301-9. PubMed PMID: 18840360. Pubmed Central PMCID: 2630775.

[27] Prieur X, Mok CY, Velagapudi VR, Nunez V, Fuentes L, Montaner D, et al. Differential lipid partitioning between adipocytes and tissue macrophages modulates macrophage lipotoxicity and M2/M1 polarization in obese mice. Diabetes. 2011 Mar;60(3): 797-809. PubMed PMID: 21266330. Pubmed Central PMCID: 3046840.

[28] Lumeng CN, DelProposto JB, Westcott DJ, Saltiel AR. Phenotypic switching of adipose tissue macrophages with obesity is generated by spatiotemporal differences in macrophage subtypes. Diabetes. 2008 Dec;57(12):3239-46. PubMed PMID: 18829989. Pubmed Central PMCID: 2584129.

[29] Li P, Lu M, Nguyen MT, Bae EJ, Chapman J, Feng D, et al. Functional heterogeneity of CD11c-positive adipose tissue macrophages in diet-induced obese mice. The Journal of biological chemistry. 2010 May 14;285(20):15333-45. PubMed PMID: 20308074. Pubmed Central PMCID: 2865288.

[30] Zhou D, Huang C, Lin Z, Zhan S, Kong L, Fang C, et al. Macrophage polarization and function with emphasis on the evolving roles of coordinated regulation of cellular signaling pathways. Cellular signalling. 2013 Nov 9;26(2):192-7. PubMed PMID: 24219909.

[31] Shi H, Kokoeva MV, Inouye K, Tzameli I, Yin H, Flier JS. TLR4 links innate immunity and fatty acid-induced insulin resistance. The Journal of clinical investigation. 2006 Nov;116(11):3015-25. PubMed PMID: 17053832. Pubmed Central PMCID: 1616196.

[32] Kang K, Reilly SM, Karabacak V, Gangl MR, Fitzgerald K, Hatano B, et al. Adipocyte-derived Th2 cytokines and myeloid PPARdelta regulate macrophage polariza-

tion and insulin sensitivity. Cell metabolism. 2008 Jun;7(6):485-95. PubMed PMID: 18522830. Pubmed Central PMCID: 2586840.

[33] Ohashi K, Parker JL, Ouchi N, Higuchi A, Vita JA, Gokce N, et al. Adiponectin promotes macrophage polarization toward an anti-inflammatory phenotype. The Journal of biological chemistry. 2010 Feb 26;285(9):6153-60. PubMed PMID: 20028977. Pubmed Central PMCID: 2825410.

[34] Rosen ED, Spiegelman BM. PPARgamma : a nuclear regulator of metabolism, differentiation, and cell growth. The Journal of biological chemistry. 2001 Oct 12;276(41): 37731-4. PubMed PMID: 11459852.

[35] Jiang C, Ting AT, Seed B. PPAR-gamma agonists inhibit production of monocyte inflammatory cytokines. Nature. 1998 Jan 1;391(6662):82-6. PubMed PMID: 9422509.

[36] Ricote M, Li AC, Willson TM, Kelly CJ, Glass CK. The peroxisome proliferator-activated receptor-gamma is a negative regulator of macrophage activation. Nature. 1998 Jan 1;391(6662):79-82. PubMed PMID: 9422508.

[37] Odegaard JI, Ricardo-Gonzalez RR, Goforth MH, Morel CR, Subramanian V, Mukundan L, et al. Macrophage-specific PPARgamma controls alternative activation and improves insulin resistance. Nature. 2007 Jun 28;447(7148):1116-20. PubMed PMID: 17515919. Pubmed Central PMCID: 2587297.

[38] Vats D, Mukundan L, Odegaard JI, Zhang L, Smith KL, Morel CR, et al. Oxidative metabolism and PGC-1beta attenuate macrophage-mediated inflammation. Cell metabolism. 2006 Jul;4(1):13-24. PubMed PMID: 16814729. Pubmed Central PMCID: 1904486.

[39] Liao X, Sharma N, Kapadia F, Zhou G, Lu Y, Hong H, et al. Kruppel-like factor 4 regulates macrophage polarization. The Journal of clinical investigation. 2011 Jul;121(7): 2736-49. PubMed PMID: 21670502. Pubmed Central PMCID: 3223832.

[40] Eguchi J, Kong X, Tenta M, Wang X, Kang S, Rosen ED. Interferon regulatory factor 4 regulates obesity-induced inflammation through regulation of adipose tissue macrophage polarization. Diabetes. 2013 Oct;62(10):3394-403. PubMed PMID: 23835343. Pubmed Central PMCID: 3781469.

[41] Huber J, Kiefer FW, Zeyda M, Ludvik B, Silberhumer GR, Prager G, et al. CC chemokine and CC chemokine receptor profiles in visceral and subcutaneous adipose tissue are altered in human obesity. The Journal of clinical endocrinology and metabolism. 2008 Aug;93(8):3215-21. PubMed PMID: 18492752.

[42] Yoshimura T, Robinson EA, Tanaka S, Appella E, Kuratsu J, Leonard EJ. Purification and amino acid analysis of two human glioma-derived monocyte chemoattractants. The Journal of experimental medicine. 1989 Apr 1;169(4):1449-59. PubMed PMID: 2926329. Pubmed Central PMCID: 2189237.

[43] Matsushima K, Larsen CG, DuBois GC, Oppenheim JJ. Purification and characterization of a novel monocyte chemotactic and activating factor produced by a human

myelomonocytic cell line. The Journal of experimental medicine. 1989 Apr 1;169(4): 1485-90. PubMed PMID: 2926331. Pubmed Central PMCID: 2189236.

[44] Rollins BJ. Chemokines. Blood. 1997 Aug 1;90(3):909-28. PubMed PMID: 9242519.

[45] Sartipy P, Loskutoff DJ. Monocyte chemoattractant protein 1 in obesity and insulin resistance. Proceedings of the National Academy of Sciences of the United States of America. 2003 Jun 10;100(12):7265-70. PubMed PMID: 12756299. Pubmed Central PMCID: 165864.

[46] Kanda H, Tateya S, Tamori Y, Kotani K, Hiasa K, Kitazawa R, et al. MCP-1 contributes to macrophage infiltration into adipose tissue, insulin resistance, and hepatic steatosis in obesity. The Journal of clinical investigation. 2006 Jun;116(6):1494-505. PubMed PMID: 16691291. Pubmed Central PMCID: 1459069. Epub 2006/05/13. eng.

[47] Weisberg SP, Hunter D, Huber R, Lemieux J, Slaymaker S, Vaddi K, et al. CCR2 modulates inflammatory and metabolic effects of high-fat feeding. The Journal of clinical investigation. 2006 Jan;116(1):115-24. PubMed PMID: 16341265. Pubmed Central PMCID: 1307559.

[48] Kamei N, Tobe K, Suzuki R, Ohsugi M, Watanabe T, Kubota N, et al. Overexpression of monocyte chemoattractant protein-1 in adipose tissues causes macrophage recruitment and insulin resistance. The Journal of biological chemistry. 2006 Sep 8;281(36): 26602-14. PubMed PMID: 16809344. Epub 2006/07/01. eng.

[49] Inouye KE, Shi H, Howard JK, Daly CH, Lord GM, Rollins BJ, et al. Absence of CC chemokine ligand 2 does not limit obesity-associated infiltration of macrophages into adipose tissue. Diabetes. 2007 Sep;56(9):2242-50. PubMed PMID: 17473219. Epub 2007/05/03. eng.

[50] Kirk EA, Sagawa ZK, McDonald TO, O'Brien KD, Heinecke JW. Monocyte chemoattractant protein deficiency fails to restrain macrophage infiltration into adipose tissue [corrected]. Diabetes. 2008 May;57(5):1254-61. PubMed PMID: 18268047. Epub 2008/02/13. eng.

[51] Jiao P, Chen Q, Shah S, Du J, Tao B, Tzameli I, et al. Obesity-related upregulation of monocyte chemotactic factors in adipocytes: involvement of nuclear factor-kappaB and c-Jun NH2-terminal kinase pathways. Diabetes. 2009 Jan;58(1):104-15. PubMed PMID: 18835938. Pubmed Central PMCID: 2606857.

[52] Murdolo G, Hammarstedt A, Sandqvist M, Schmelz M, Herder C, Smith U, et al. Monocyte chemoattractant protein-1 in subcutaneous abdominal adipose tissue: characterization of interstitial concentration and regulation of gene expression by insulin. The Journal of clinical endocrinology and metabolism. 2007 Jul;92(7):2688-95. PubMed PMID: 17456576.

[53] Westerbacka J, Corner A, Kolak M, Makkonen J, Turpeinen U, Hamsten A, et al. Insulin regulation of MCP-1 in human adipose tissue of obese and lean women. Ameri-

can journal of physiology Endocrinology and metabolism. 2008 May;294(5):E841-5. PubMed PMID: 18270300.

[54] Surmi BK, Webb CD, Ristau AC, Hasty AH. Absence of macrophage inflammatory protein-1{alpha} does not impact macrophage accumulation in adipose tissue of diet-induced obese mice. American journal of physiology Endocrinology and metabolism. 2010 Sep;299(3):E437-45. PubMed PMID: 20551286. Pubmed Central PMCID: 2944285.

[55] Keophiphath M, Rouault C, Divoux A, Clement K, Lacasa D. CCL5 promotes macrophage recruitment and survival in human adipose tissue. Arteriosclerosis, thrombosis, and vascular biology. 2010 Jan;30(1):39-45. PubMed PMID: 19893003.

[56] Eriksson EE. Mechanisms of leukocyte recruitment to atherosclerotic lesions: future prospects. Current opinion in lipidology. 2004 Oct;15(5):553-8. PubMed PMID: 15361791.

[57] Zernecke A, Shagdarsuren E, Weber C. Chemokines in atherosclerosis: an update. Arteriosclerosis, thrombosis, and vascular biology. 2008 Nov;28(11):1897-908. PubMed PMID: 18566299.

[58] Kitade H, Sawamoto K, Nagashimada M, Inoue H, Yamamoto Y, Sai Y, et al. CCR5 plays a critical role in obesity-induced adipose tissue inflammation and insulin resistance by regulating both macrophage recruitment and M1/M2 status. Diabetes. 2012 Jul;61(7):1680-90. PubMed PMID: 22474027. Pubmed Central PMCID: 3379680.

[59] Samuelsson B, Dahlen SE, Lindgren JA, Rouzer CA, Serhan CN. Leukotrienes and lipoxins: structures, biosynthesis, and biological effects. Science. 1987 Sep 4;237(4819):1171-6. PubMed PMID: 2820055.

[60] Haeggstrom JZ. Leukotriene A4 hydrolase/aminopeptidase, the gatekeeper of chemotactic leukotriene B4 biosynthesis. The Journal of biological chemistry. 2004 Dec 3;279(49):50639-42. PubMed PMID: 15339917.

[61] Yokomizo T, Izumi T, Chang K, Takuwa Y, Shimizu T. A G-protein-coupled receptor for leukotriene B4 that mediates chemotaxis. Nature. 1997 Jun 5;387(6633):620-4. PubMed PMID: 9177352.

[62] Chou RC, Kim ND, Sadik CD, Seung E, Lan Y, Byrne MH, et al. Lipid-cytokine-chemokine cascade drives neutrophil recruitment in a murine model of inflammatory arthritis. Immunity. 2010 Aug 27;33(2):266-78. PubMed PMID: 20727790. Pubmed Central PMCID: 3155777.

[63] Haribabu B, Verghese MW, Steeber DA, Sellars DD, Bock CB, Snyderman R. Targeted disruption of the leukotriene B(4) receptor in mice reveals its role in inflammation and platelet-activating factor-induced anaphylaxis. The Journal of experimental medicine. 2000 Aug 7;192(3):433-8. PubMed PMID: 10934231. Pubmed Central PMCID: 2193219.

[64] Subbarao K, Jala VR, Mathis S, Suttles J, Zacharias W, Ahamed J, et al. Role of leukotriene B4 receptors in the development of atherosclerosis: potential mechanisms. Arteriosclerosis, thrombosis, and vascular biology. 2004 Feb;24(2):369-75. PubMed PMID: 14656734.

[65] Tager AM, Dufour JH, Goodarzi K, Bercury SD, von Andrian UH, Luster AD. BLTR mediates leukotriene B(4)-induced chemotaxis and adhesion and plays a dominant role in eosinophil accumulation in a murine model of peritonitis. The Journal of experimental medicine. 2000 Aug 7;192(3):439-46. PubMed PMID: 10934232. Pubmed Central PMCID: 2193216.

[66] Back M, Bu DX, Branstrom R, Sheikine Y, Yan ZQ, Hansson GK. Leukotriene B4 signaling through NF-kappaB-dependent BLT1 receptors on vascular smooth muscle cells in atherosclerosis and intimal hyperplasia. Proceedings of the National Academy of Sciences of the United States of America. 2005 Nov 29;102(48):17501-6. PubMed PMID: 16293697. Pubmed Central PMCID: 1297663.

[67] Back M, Sultan A, Ovchinnikova O, Hansson GK. 5-Lipoxygenase-activating protein: a potential link between innate and adaptive immunity in atherosclerosis and adipose tissue inflammation. Circulation research. 2007 Apr 13;100(7):946-9. PubMed PMID: 17379835.

[68] Horrillo R, Gonzalez-Periz A, Martinez-Clemente M, Lopez-Parra M, Ferre N, Titos E, et al. 5-lipoxygenase activating protein signals adipose tissue inflammation and lipid dysfunction in experimental obesity. Journal of immunology. 2010 Apr 1;184(7): 3978-87. PubMed PMID: 20207999.

[69] Chakrabarti SK, Wen Y, Dobrian AD, Cole BK, Ma Q, Pei H, et al. Evidence for activation of inflammatory lipoxygenase pathways in visceral adipose tissue of obese Zucker rats. American journal of physiology Endocrinology and metabolism. 2011 Jan;300(1):E175-87. PubMed PMID: 20978234. Pubmed Central PMCID: 3023204.

[70] Spite M, Hellmann J, Tang Y, Mathis SP, Kosuri M, Bhatnagar A, et al. Deficiency of the leukotriene B4 receptor, BLT-1, protects against systemic insulin resistance in diet-induced obesity. Journal of immunology. 2011 Aug 15;187(4):1942-9. PubMed PMID: 21742977. Pubmed Central PMCID: 3150353.

[71] D'Haese JG, Demir IE, Friess H, Ceyhan GO. Fractalkine/CX3CR1: why a single chemokine-receptor duo bears a major and unique therapeutic potential. Expert opinion on therapeutic targets. 2010 Feb;14(2):207-19. PubMed PMID: 20055718.

[72] Bazan JF, Bacon KB, Hardiman G, Wang W, Soo K, Rossi D, et al. A new class of membrane-bound chemokine with a CX3C motif. Nature. 1997 Feb 13;385(6617): 640-4. PubMed PMID: 9024663.

[73] Imai T, Hieshima K, Haskell C, Baba M, Nagira M, Nishimura M, et al. Identification and molecular characterization of fractalkine receptor CX3CR1, which mediates both

leukocyte migration and adhesion. Cell. 1997 Nov 14;91(4):521-30. PubMed PMID: 9390561.

[74] Lee SJ, Namkoong S, Kim YM, Kim CK, Lee H, Ha KS, et al. Fractalkine stimulates angiogenesis by activating the Raf-1/MEK/ERK-and PI3K/Akt/eNOS-dependent signal pathways. American journal of physiology Heart and circulatory physiology. 2006 Dec;291(6):H2836-46. PubMed PMID: 16877565.

[75] Saederup N, Chan L, Lira SA, Charo IF. Fractalkine deficiency markedly reduces macrophage accumulation and atherosclerotic lesion formation in CCR2-/-mice: evidence for independent chemokine functions in atherogenesis. Circulation. 2008 Apr 1;117(13):1642-8. PubMed PMID: 18165355. Pubmed Central PMCID: 3589525.

[76] Landsman L, Bar-On L, Zernecke A, Kim KW, Krauthgamer R, Shagdarsuren E, et al. CX3CR1 is required for monocyte homeostasis and atherogenesis by promoting cell survival. Blood. 2009 Jan 22;113(4):963-72. PubMed PMID: 18971423.

[77] Digby JE, McNeill E, Dyar OJ, Lam V, Greaves DR, Choudhury RP. Anti-inflammatory effects of nicotinic acid in adipocytes demonstrated by suppression of fractalkine, RANTES, and MCP-1 and upregulation of adiponectin. Atherosclerosis. 2010 Mar; 209(1):89-95. PubMed PMID: 19781706. Pubmed Central PMCID: 2839075.

[78] Lesnik P, Haskell CA, Charo IF. Decreased atherosclerosis in CX3CR1-/-mice reveals a role for fractalkine in atherogenesis. The Journal of clinical investigation. 2003 Feb; 111(3):333-40. PubMed PMID: 12569158. Pubmed Central PMCID: 151849.

[79] Shah R, Lu Y, Hinkle CC, McGillicuddy FC, Kim R, Hannenhalli S, et al. Gene profiling of human adipose tissue during evoked inflammation in vivo. Diabetes. 2009 Oct; 58(10):2211-9. PubMed PMID: 19581417. Pubmed Central PMCID: 2750231.

[80] Shah R, Hinkle CC, Ferguson JF, Mehta NN, Li M, Qu L, et al. Fractalkine is a novel human adipochemokine associated with type 2 diabetes. Diabetes. 2011 May;60(5): 1512-8. PubMed PMID: 21525510. Pubmed Central PMCID: 3292325.

[81] Hromas R, Broxmeyer HE, Kim C, Nakshatri H, Christopherson K, 2nd, Azam M, et al. Cloning of BRAK, a novel divergent CXC chemokine preferentially expressed in normal versus malignant cells. Biochemical and biophysical research communications. 1999 Feb 24;255(3):703-6. PubMed PMID: 10049774.

[82] Sleeman MA, Fraser JK, Murison JG, Kelly SL, Prestidge RL, Palmer DJ, et al. B cell- and monocyte-activating chemokine (BMAC), a novel non-ELR alpha-chemokine. International immunology. 2000 May;12(5):677-89. PubMed PMID: 10784614.

[83] Frederick MJ, Henderson Y, Xu X, Deavers MT, Sahin AA, Wu H, et al. In vivo expression of the novel CXC chemokine BRAK in normal and cancerous human tissue. The American journal of pathology. 2000 Jun;156(6):1937-50. PubMed PMID: 10854217. Pubmed Central PMCID: 1850081.

[84] Cao X, Zhang W, Wan T, He L, Chen T, Yuan Z, et al. Molecular cloning and characterization of a novel CXC chemokine macrophage inflammatory protein-2 gamma

chemoattractant for human neutrophils and dendritic cells. Journal of immunology. 2000 Sep 1;165(5):2588-95. PubMed PMID: 10946286.

[85] Shellenberger TD, Wang M, Gujrati M, Jayakumar A, Strieter RM, Burdick MD, et al. BRAK/CXCL14 is a potent inhibitor of angiogenesis and a chemotactic factor for immature dendritic cells. Cancer research. 2004 Nov 15;64(22):8262-70. PubMed PMID: 15548693.

[86] Shurin GV, Ferris RL, Tourkova IL, Perez L, Lokshin A, Balkir L, et al. Loss of new chemokine CXCL14 in tumor tissue is associated with low infiltration by dendritic cells (DC), while restoration of human CXCL14 expression in tumor cells causes attraction of DC both in vitro and in vivo. Journal of immunology. 2005 May 1;174(9): 5490-8. PubMed PMID: 15843547.

[87] Schaerli P, Willimann K, Ebert LM, Walz A, Moser B. Cutaneous CXCL14 targets blood precursors to epidermal niches for Langerhans cell differentiation. Immunity. 2005 Sep;23(3):331-42. PubMed PMID: 16169505.

[88] Nara N, Nakayama Y, Okamoto S, Tamura H, Kiyono M, Muraoka M, et al. Disruption of CXC motif chemokine ligand-14 in mice ameliorates obesity-induced insulin resistance. The Journal of biological chemistry. 2007 Oct 19;282(42):30794-803. PubMed PMID: 17724031.

[89] Ashkar S, Weber GF, Panoutsakopoulou V, Sanchirico ME, Jansson M, Zawaideh S, et al. Eta-1 (osteopontin): an early component of type-1 (cell-mediated) immunity. Science. 2000 Feb 4;287(5454):860-4. PubMed PMID: 10657301.

[90] Reinholt FP, Hultenby K, Oldberg A, Heinegard D. Osteopontin--a possible anchor of osteoclasts to bone. Proceedings of the National Academy of Sciences of the United States of America. 1990 Jun;87(12):4473-5. PubMed PMID: 1693772. Pubmed Central PMCID: 54137.

[91] Giachelli CM, Lombardi D, Johnson RJ, Murry CE, Almeida M. Evidence for a role of osteopontin in macrophage infiltration in response to pathological stimuli in vivo. The American journal of pathology. 1998 Feb;152(2):353-8. PubMed PMID: 9466560. Pubmed Central PMCID: 1857977.

[92] Nystrom T, Duner P, Hultgardh-Nilsson A. A constitutive endogenous osteopontin production is important for macrophage function and differentiation. Experimental cell research. 2007 Apr 1;313(6):1149-60. PubMed PMID: 17306792.

[93] Murry CE, Giachelli CM, Schwartz SM, Vracko R. Macrophages express osteopontin during repair of myocardial necrosis. The American journal of pathology. 1994 Dec; 145(6):1450-62. PubMed PMID: 7992848. Pubmed Central PMCID: 1887495.

[94] Denhardt DT, Giachelli CM, Rittling SR. Role of osteopontin in cellular signaling and toxicant injury. Annual review of pharmacology and toxicology. 2001;41:723-49. PubMed PMID: 11264474.

[95] Denhardt DT, Noda M, O'Regan AW, Pavlin D, Berman JS. Osteopontin as a means to cope with environmental insults: regulation of inflammation, tissue remodeling, and cell survival. The Journal of clinical investigation. 2001 May;107(9):1055-61. PubMed PMID: 11342566. Pubmed Central PMCID: 209291.

[96] Nomiyama T, Perez-Tilve D, Ogawa D, Gizard F, Zhao Y, Heywood EB, et al. Osteopontin mediates obesity-induced adipose tissue macrophage infiltration and insulin resistance in mice. The Journal of clinical investigation. 2007 Oct;117(10):2877-88. PubMed PMID: 17823662. Pubmed Central PMCID: 1964510.

[97] Miyazaki T, Hirokami Y, Matsuhashi N, Takatsuka H, Naito M. Increased susceptibility of thymocytes to apoptosis in mice lacking AIM, a novel murine macrophage-derived soluble factor belonging to the scavenger receptor cysteine-rich domain superfamily. The Journal of experimental medicine. 1999 Jan 18;189(2):413-22. PubMed PMID: 9892623. Pubmed Central PMCID: 2192994.

[98] Kurokawa J, Arai S, Nakashima K, Nagano H, Nishijima A, Miyata K, et al. Macrophage-derived AIM is endocytosed into adipocytes and decreases lipid droplets via inhibition of fatty acid synthase activity. Cell metabolism. 2010 Jun 9;11(6):479-92. PubMed PMID: 20519120.

[99] Joseph SB, Bradley MN, Castrillo A, Bruhn KW, Mak PA, Pei L, et al. LXR-dependent gene expression is important for macrophage survival and the innate immune response. Cell. 2004 Oct 15;119(2):299-309. PubMed PMID: 15479645.

[100] Valledor AF, Hsu LC, Ogawa S, Sawka-Verhelle D, Karin M, Glass CK. Activation of liver X receptors and retinoid X receptors prevents bacterial-induced macrophage apoptosis. Proceedings of the National Academy of Sciences of the United States of America. 2004 Dec 21;101(51):17813-8. PubMed PMID: 15601766. Pubmed Central PMCID: 539759.

[101] Gebe JA, Kiener PA, Ring HZ, Li X, Francke U, Aruffo A. Molecular cloning, mapping to human chromosome 1 q21-q23, and cell binding characteristics of Spalpha, a new member of the scavenger receptor cysteine-rich (SRCR) family of proteins. The Journal of biological chemistry. 1997 Mar 7;272(10):6151-8. PubMed PMID: 9045627.

[102] Kim WK, Hwang HR, Kim do H, Lee PY, In YJ, Ryu HY, et al. Glycoproteomic analysis of plasma from patients with atopic dermatitis: CD5L and ApoE as potential biomarkers. Experimental & molecular medicine. 2008 Dec 31;40(6):677-85. PubMed PMID: 19116453. Pubmed Central PMCID: 2679343.

[103] Gray J, Chattopadhyay D, Beale GS, Patman GL, Miele L, King BP, et al. A proteomic strategy to identify novel serum biomarkers for liver cirrhosis and hepatocellular cancer in individuals with fatty liver disease. BMC cancer. 2009;9:271. PubMed PMID: 19656391. Pubmed Central PMCID: 2729079.

[104] Kurokawa J, Nagano H, Ohara O, Kubota N, Kadowaki T, Arai S, et al. Apoptosis inhibitor of macrophage (AIM) is required for obesity-associated recruitment of in-

flammatory macrophages into adipose tissue. Proceedings of the National Academy of Sciences of the United States of America. 2011 Jul 19;108(29):12072-7. PubMed PMID: 21730133. Pubmed Central PMCID: 3141977.

[105] Schaffler A, Scholmerich J, Salzberger B. Adipose tissue as an immunological organ: Toll-like receptors, C1q/TNFs and CTRPs. Trends in immunology. 2007 Sep;28(9): 393-9. PubMed PMID: 17681884.

[106] Calandra T, Bernhagen J, Mitchell RA, Bucala R. The macrophage is an important and previously unrecognized source of macrophage migration inhibitory factor. The Journal of experimental medicine. 1994 Jun 1;179(6):1895-902. PubMed PMID: 8195715. Pubmed Central PMCID: 2191507.

[107] Baugh JA, Bucala R. Macrophage migration inhibitory factor. Critical care medicine. 2002 Jan;30(1 Supp):S27-S35. PubMed PMID: 11891404.

[108] Calandra T, Roger T. Macrophage migration inhibitory factor: a regulator of innate immunity. Nature reviews Immunology. 2003 Oct;3(10):791-800. PubMed PMID: 14502271.

[109] Gregory JL, Morand EF, McKeown SJ, Ralph JA, Hall P, Yang YH, et al. Macrophage migration inhibitory factor induces macrophage recruitment via CC chemokine ligand 2. Journal of immunology. 2006 Dec 1;177(11):8072-9. PubMed PMID: 17114481.

[110] Toso C, Emamaullee JA, Merani S, Shapiro AM. The role of macrophage migration inhibitory factor on glucose metabolism and diabetes. Diabetologia. 2008 Nov;51(11): 1937-46. PubMed PMID: 18612626.

[111] Bernhagen J, Krohn R, Lue H, Gregory JL, Zernecke A, Koenen RR, et al. MIF is a noncognate ligand of CXC chemokine receptors in inflammatory and atherogenic cell recruitment. Nature medicine. 2007 May;13(5):587-96. PubMed PMID: 17435771.

[112] Lue H, Dewor M, Leng L, Bucala R, Bernhagen J. Activation of the JNK signalling pathway by macrophage migration inhibitory factor (MIF) and dependence on CXCR4 and CD74. Cellular signalling. 2011 Jan;23(1):135-44. PubMed PMID: 20807568. Pubmed Central PMCID: 3586206.

[113] Fan H, Hall P, Santos LL, Gregory JL, Fingerle-Rowson G, Bucala R, et al. Macrophage migration inhibitory factor and CD74 regulate macrophage chemotactic responses via MAPK and Rho GTPase. Journal of immunology. 2011 Apr 15;186(8): 4915-24. PubMed PMID: 21411731. Pubmed Central PMCID: 3388798.

[114] Finucane OM, Reynolds CM, McGillicuddy FC, Roche HM. Insights into the role of macrophage migration inhibitory factor in obesity and insulin resistance. The Proceedings of the Nutrition Society. 2012 Nov;71(4):622-33. PubMed PMID: 22914223.

[115] Conine SJ, Cross JV. MIF deficiency does not alter glucose homeostasis or adipose tissue inflammatory cell infiltrates during diet-induced obesity. Obesity. 2013 Jun 26. PubMed PMID: 23804488.

Chapter 7

Thyrotropin-Releasing Hormone (TRH) a Small Molecule in Pancreas Promotes Insulin Producing Cell Proliferation

John Z.Q . Luo, Souriya Vang, Zhao Ting,
Ivor Jackson and LuGuang Luo

Additional information is available at the end of the chapter

http://dx.doi.org/10.5772/57550

1. Introduction

Neural tripeptide amide L-pyroglutamyl-L-histidyl-L-prolineamide (L-PHP, Thyrotropin-releasing hormone, TRH) is a fine molecular peptide that was first identified in the Central Nervous System (CNS) and discovered in many other regions of body later as a neuropeptide hormone or neuromodulator [1]. L-PHP stimulates the thyroid stimulating hormone (TSH) after it is released from the hypothalamic nerve in the median eminence. L-PHP was named as its functional action-TRH [2]. Beyond neuronal tissue, expression of L-PHP was also found in the pancreatic islets where it identifies to the Langerhans-insulin-producing beta cells [3]. However, L-PHP expression and production is significantly different from its production in the nervous system; it is primarily expressed during the early developmental period in rat [4] and human fetal pancreatic tissue [4]. L-PHP stimulates glucagon release and inhibits other pancreatic secretion other than TSH [5]. In this review, based on evidence found in L-PHP gene knockout animal models and its function in regulating insulin release in pancreatic tissue [6], L-PHP may play an important role in carbohydrate metabolism and pancreatic L-PHP disruption may lead to the development of diabetes mellitus.

Expression of L-PHP in the pancreas: L-PHP is expressed in the insulin granules of β cells in pancreatic islets, [7] with high levels during the neonatal period but significantly decreased as postnatal development progresses [4]. A Comparison with L-PHP expression, in the primary transition period between E12 and E14, shows insulin secretion in both rat and mouse while L-PHP remains unexpressed[4, 8]. During this period, insulin stained cells do not express any Rab3A, SNAP-25 (two molecules important for the control of insulin secretion) nor Glut 2 and

granules resemble β cells. However, at E16, L-PHP expression was found and thereafter, high expression of molecules such as Glut2 and Pdx-1, which are necessary for insulin production, maturation and full insulin cell function, were found in the insulin and L-PHP positive cells. L-PHP's significant expression coincides with factors for insulin production, maturation and insulin cell development suggesting that L-PHP is critical for insulin cells as they become functionally mature during early development.

2. Effects of L-PHP on pancreatic insulin secretion

Beyond regulating TSH, L-PHP is also found to be involved in the regulation of neuronal growth [9], facilitating spinal cord injury recovery [10], appetite control [11], and alcohol consumption [12]. The most important role of L-PHP is considered to be its regulation of blood glucose levels *in vivo*, presumably *via* the CNS [6, 13-16]. L-PHP's anti-hyperglycemia function was identified by eliminating pituitary-thyroid axis by a hypophysectomy, which also eliminated other hormones released from pituitary, and suggests its anti-hyperglycemia function beyond its activation in CNS [17]. In another experiment, pancreatic beta cells were destroyed by Streptozotocin and CNS administration of L-PHP failed to reverse high blood glucose, supporting this notion of function outside of CNS activation. L-PHP regulating blood glucose may have a direct effect in pancreatic beta cell instead of *via* CNS or thyroid hormone, which was supported by application of thyroid hormone in hypothyroidism of hyperglycemic animal but did not reverse high blood glucose. Blood glucagon and insulin level was increased by intravenous injection of L-PHP in rabbit [18] and cultured fetal islet identified L-PHP expression by a quantitative analysis [19] which supports the possibility of L-PHP's direct effect on pancreatic beta cell function.

Pancreatic L-PHP can stimulate pancreatic endocrine function and/or endocrine cell development. The mechanisms as to how L-PHP regulates pancreatic β-cell development have not been identified. Gathering evidence from *in vivo* and *in vitro*, we propose that L-PHP may modulate insulin secretion directly when glucose stimulates β-cell, which was demonstrated in isolated perfusion of fresh islets [20] and islet cell lines (Fig. 1). The mechanisms may relate to L-PHP regulating glucagon-containing (alpha) cell secretion resulting in eliminating somatostatin (r-cells) and inhibiting insulin production. A clinical study in hyperparathyroidism patients showed that L-PHP application to these patients significantly elevated serum levels of insulin and glucagon and it also had a dose-dependent inhibition of carbachol-stimulated amylase secretion, suggesting a role for L-PHP in the paracrine regulation of exocrine as well as endocrine pancreatic secretion.

L-PHP protects pancreatic tissue from damage and toxins like the reduction of glycodeoxycholic acid. Evidence suggests that L-PHP plays a critical role in β-cell maturation. During the phase of pancreatic development, which includes high levels of L-PHP expression in early pancreatic β-cell development, dexamethasone treatment eliminated the L-PHP peak and resulted in retarded β-cell development [21]. Also, newborn rats were found to have reduced L-PHP levels due to maternal diabetes caused by streptozotocin (STZ) injection [22]. The

http://dx.doi.org/10.5772/57550

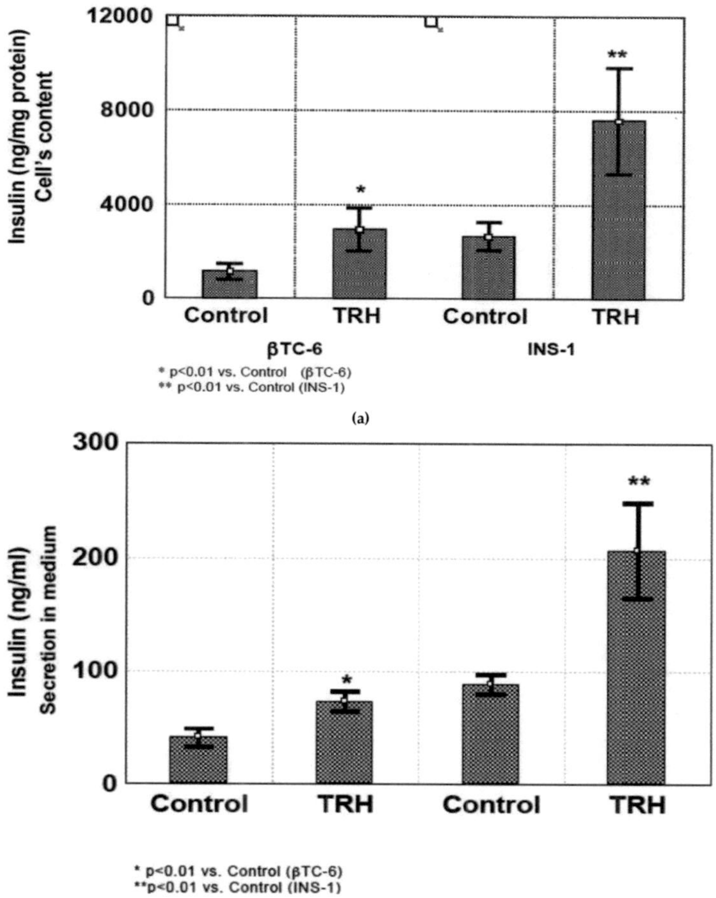

Figure 1. Insulin levels in βTC-6 (a mouse derived pancreatic β cell line) cell extracts and medium after exposure to TRH Cells were cultured for 24 hours with or without TRH (n=6 each group). Culture Medium was collected and harvested cells were extracted by 5% TCA. Insulin content and secretion were measured by ELISA. Insulin content was normalized relative to protein concentration (mg/ml) in the cell extracts. L-PHP treated cells contained greater levels of insulin in cell extracts A and culture medium B vs controls. (From reference #25, with permission)

observation of ten-fold lower L-PHP in pups of diabetic rat followed by a postnatal day 5 elevation of L-PHP reducing blood glucose levels [22] suggest that L-PHP expression during β-cell development is important and it may prevent diabetes from developing in later life.

The L-PHP receptor consists of two major sub-types (R1 and R2, recently identified third type). Using RT-PCR, receptor R1 is identified as expressed in HIT-T15 (HIT) cells, a hamster clonal ß-cell line [23], and mouse pancreatic islets, but expression of R2 is not found. R2 was identified as expressed predominantly in the CNS, but not other tissue. By northern blot analysis it was found that R1 in pancreas is of 3.7-kb size and shares 93.3% homology with that in the pituitary. Evaluation of R1 function by receptor affinity found various kDa values in ß –cells [23]. ß –cell intracellular calcium concentration was significantly increased by L-PHP and removal of extracellular calcium does not change this effect [24]. Our group work has shown

R1 expression in rat-derived β-cell lines as well as whole pancreas that included nonislet tissue [25]. R1 receptor was also found to associate with EGF receptor function called cross linking [25] (Fig. 2).

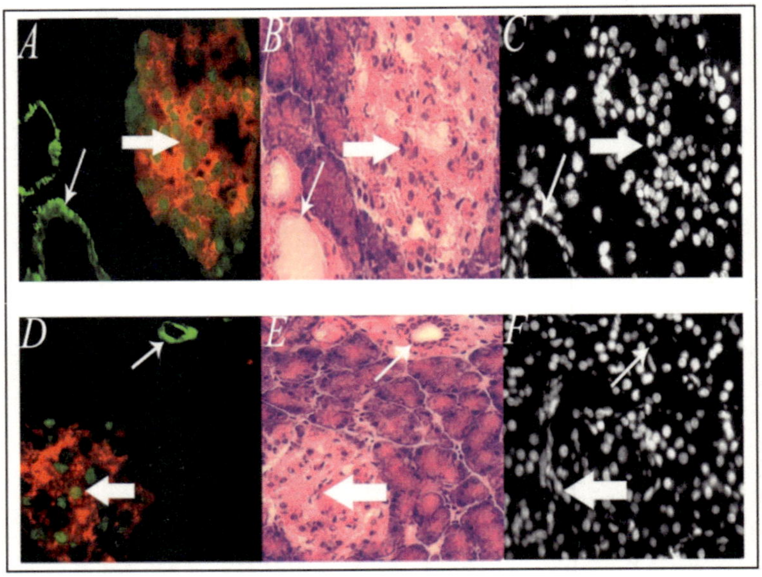

Figure 2. In situ hybridization of L-PHP-receptor-1(R1) in rat pancreas A. and D. Dual fluorescent image of rat pancreas. Red indicates insulin immuno-fluorescence; Green indicates R1 in situ hybridization. B. and E show H&E staining for tissue morphology, C and F show dapi for nuclei staining. The large arrows indicate the yellow color, a mixture of green and red represents colocalization of insulin and R1 in islet and the small white arrows indicate the positive staining of R1 in epithelial A. B. and ductal D. E. (From reference #25, with permission)

3. Regulation of L-PHP in the pancreas

In vitro studies have shown that L-PHP is stimulated by glucose and suppressed by insulin release. Cellular cAMP production regulated by somatostatin may involve glucose and insulin regulation of L-PHP [26, 27]. We hypothesize that there is an α-β-γ integrating system, which releases insulin-L-PHP-somatostatin coordinated in respond to glucose challenge in islet. To support this hypothesis, it needs further study but evidence in that tissue cultures of pure β cell do not function as well as an entire islet may be part of the support.

4. L-PHP alteration of gene expression modifys microenvironment within the pancreas

Pancreatic microenvironment alteration by L-PHP has been reported [28]. The findings show that multiple functional genes in rat pancreas were influenced by L-PHP *in vivo*. A total of 60

http://dx.doi.org/10.5772/57550

genes are found to be regulated by L-PHP, 29 genes in the pancreas and 31 genes in rat derived pancreatic β-cell line, INS-1 cells. These genes include Ca2+channel enhancers (Ca2+/calmodulin-dependent protein kinase, type I and II), G-protein coupling receptor related genes (GPCR kinase 4 and 5, transducin-β 1 subunit,Arrestin-β1, transducin-β1), Protein kinases (serine/threonine kinase-3,PKC β, PCTAIRE-3, v-mos), proliferation or differentiation signal transduction related genes (MAPK3, growth factor receptor-bound protein 2, n-myc, GAP-43) and down-regulated pro-apoptotic Bax gene. Genes relative to insulin secretion are significantly increased by L-PHP including N-methyl-D-aspartate receptor-2A, GABA-A receptor, RAB2, Ras-related GTPase and ADP ribosylation factor 1 and 5. The differential gene expression between β-cells and total pancreatic tissue in response to L-PHP shows that of the 36 genes that are initiated and 36 genes that are turned off relative to signal transduction. In rat pancreas 6 genes were initiated and 14 genes were turned off, with one initiating the anti-apoptotic BcLX gene. While in rat INS-1 β cell line only 4 genes were initiated and 4 genes turned off from the 34 signal transduction genes. These significant variations between pure β-cell and entire pancreatic tissue indicate that L-PHP can regulate β-cell function by directly working on β-cells or by indirectly altering pancreatic microenvironment to maintain and facilitate β-cell response to glucose resulting in a balance *in vivo* of glucose metabolism.

5. Regulation of β-cell proliferation by signal pathways from L-PHP to growth hormone activity in pancreatic islet

L-PHP has been reported to stimulate R1 and dissociate the GPCR complex, activating protein kinase C [29] and mitogen-activated protein kinase (MAPK) [29] in both a PKC-dependent and a PKC-independent manner in the neuronal cell lines [30]. These effects may involve activation of tyrosine kinase, which leads to the activation of Ras and MAPK cascade. The signaling pathways initiating from G-coupled L-PHP receptor in activating MAPK may overlap with the receptor tyrosine kinases activating the Ras-MAPK cascade [31, 32]. There is evidence that L-PHP and EGF have overlapping activities [33] leading to the stimulation of tyrosine phosphorylation of EGF receptors in GH3 cells, a pituitary cell line [34]. L-PHP-induced EGF receptor phosphorylation led to the recruitment of adapter protein Grb2 and Shc in GH3 cells. The hypothesis that L-PHP would activate EGF receptors in β cells through multiple pathways is tested, and data indicated that L-PHP trans-activates EGF receptors through several intra- and extracellular pathways, which are distinguished from pituitary-derived cell lines. R1 can initiate multiple signal transduction pathways to activate the epidermal growth factor (EGF) receptor in pancreatic β cells [35]. By initiating R1 G-protein-coupled receptor (GPCR) and dissociated αβγ complex, L-PHP (200nM) activates tyrosine residues at Tyr845, (a known target for Src) and Tyr1068 in the EGF receptor complex in an immortalized mouse β-cell line, βTC-6. Through manipulating the activation of Src, PKC and heparin-binding EGF-like growth factor (HB-EGF) with corresponding individual inhibitors and activators, multiple signal transduction pathways linking L-PHP to EGF receptors in βTC-6 cell lines have been revealed. The pathways include the activation of Src kinase and the release of heparin-binding EGF as a consequence of MMP3 activation. Alternatively, L-PHP inhibited PKC activity by reducing

EGF receptor serine/threonine phosphorylation, thereby enhancing tyrosine phosphorylation. L-PHP receptor activation of Src may have a central role in mediating the effects of L-PHP on the EGF receptor (Fig. 3). The activation of the EGF receptor by L-PHP in multiple circumstances may have important implications for pancreatic β cell biology. Since EGF receptor expression has been found to have a high activity during the embryonic developmental period [4, 36], the possibility exists that L-PHP activation of EGF receptors in pancreatic β cells may play a role in β-cell development.

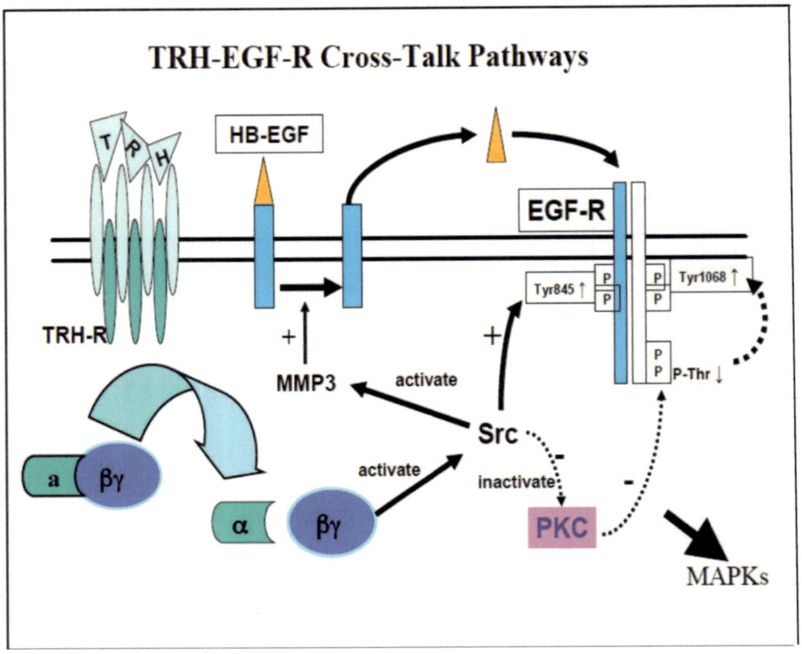

Figure 3. The scheme summarized the mechanism of L-PHP cross talk with EGF receptor in pancreatic β cells. L-PHP binds to its receptor and dissociates GPCR αβγ complex into α and βγ units. The βγ unit activation of the Src kinase directly results in phosphorylation of EGF receptor Tyr 845. In addition, Src indirectly stimulates Tyr 845 phosphorylation by activation of MMP3 to release heparin-binding EGF. Meanwhile, activation of Src kinase inhibition of PKC results in reducing serine/threonine phosphorylation which blocks off the inhibition of serine/threonine phosphorylation on tyrosine phosphorylation and indirectly activates Tyr 1068 phosphorylation in EGF receptor. L-PHP activation of EGF receptor phosphorylation results in the activation of cellular signal pathways such as MAPKs. The activation of Src may have a central role in mediating the effects of L-PHP on the EGF receptor. (R=receptor; _____=activation;------=suppression) (From reference #35, with permission)

6. Conclusions

The small sized L-PHP neuropeptide may play a significant role in direct regulation of pancreatic β-cell function and, through modulation of pancreatic microenvironment, support β-cell survival. The role of L-PHP may be similar to that of the gut peptide GLP-1, that increases β-cell regeneration, but may also have a role in inducing adult stem cell differentiation into functional β-cells during pancreatic tissue injury, which may be significant for diabetic therapy.

7. Future directions

Rat islet cell function can be recovered 90-95% from a pancreatectomy after application of glucagon-like peptide 1(GLP-1) [38]. This β-cell regeneration from damaged rat pancreas has also been mimicked by STZ damaged rat pancreas following administration of L-PHP [39]. However, human islet β-cell regeneration may differ from rat and it may require a totally different microenvironment. In order to initiate human islet β-cell functional recovery from damage or loss, pancreatic stem cells or stem cells from other tissue, such as bone marrow, must be able to in vivo differentiate into multiple types of endocrine cells ($\alpha\beta\gamma$) to reconstitute a new endocrine system in response to glucose challenge. Initiating L-PHP generation *in vivo* or administration from *in vitro* may be a way to approach this goal. Before the application of this peptide, a series of studies must be performed 1) to prove L-PHP can induce stem cells in the pancreatic environment to differentiate into β-cells and 2) L-PHP can induce other islet endocrine cells, such as α and γ cells, to support and regulate β-cell function, even β-cell regeneration. The current evidence from in vivo animal models and in vitro is very promising and encouraging; still multiple steps are needed before L-PHP can be applied in human diabetic therapy.

Acknowledgements

This work was partially supported by Roger Williams Hospital Research fund, and NIH Grant Number 1R01DK097380-01A1 from National Institute of Diabetes and Digestive and Kidney Diseases (NIDDK) and National Institute of General Medical Sciences (NIGMS). Its contents are solely the responsibility of the authors and do not necessarily represent the official views of the NIH.

Author details

John Z.Q . Luo[1], Souriya Vang[2], Zhao Ting[2], Ivor Jackson[1] and LuGuang Luo[2*]

*Address all correspondence to: lluo@rwmc.org

1 Brown Alpert Medical School, Rhode Island, USA

2 Department Research, Center of Stem Cell Research, Roger Williams Hospital Providence, Rhode Island, USA

References

[1] Engler D, Scanlon MF, Jackson IM. Thyrotropin-releasing hormone in the systemic circulation of the neonatal rat is derived from the pancreas and other extraneural tissues. J Clin Invest 1981; 67: 800-8.

[2] Reichlin S, Saperstein R, Jackson IM, Boyd AE 3rd, Patel Y. Hypothalamic hormones. Annu Rev Physiol 1976; 38: 389-424.

[3] Wu P, Jackson IM. Identification, characterization and localization of thyrotropin-releasing hormone precursor peptides in perinatal rat pancreas. Regul Pept 1988; 22(4): 347-60.

[4] Basmaciogullari A, Cras-Meneur C, Czernichow P, Scharfmann R. Pancreatic pattern of expression of thyrotropin-releasing hormone during rat embryonic development. J Endocrinol 2000; 166: 481-8.

[5] Yamagishi K. Pancreatic exocrine and endocrine functions stimulated with secretin and thyrotropin-releasing hormone in patients with hyperparathyroidism. Nihon Geka Gakkai Zasshi 1992; 93(5): 494-504.

[6] Yamada M, Saga Y, Shibusawa N, *et al.* Tertiary hypothyroidism and hyperglycemia in mice with targeted disruption of the thyrotropin-releasing hormone gene. Proc Natl Acad Sci USA 1997; 94: 10862-7.

[7] Fragner P, Ladram A, Aratan de Leon S. Triiodothyronine down-regulates thyrotropin-releasing hormone (TRH) synthesis and decreases pTRH-(160-169) and insulin releases from fetal rat islets in culture. Endocrinology 1999; 140(9): 4113-9.

[8] Yamaoka T, Itakura M. Development of pancreatic islets (review). Int J Mol Med 1999; 3: 247-61.

[9] Koenig ML, Sgarlat CM, Yourick DL, Long JB, Meyerhoff JL. *In vitro* neuroprotection against glutamate-induced toxicity by pGlu-Glu-Pro-NH(2) (EEP). Peptides 2001; 22: 2091-7.

[10] Behrmann DL, Bresnahan JC, Beattie MS. Modeling of acute spinal cord injury in the rat: neuroprotection and enhanced recovery with methylprednisolone, U-74006F and YM-14673. Exp Neurol. 1994;126: 61-75.

[11] Stanley SA, Small CJ, Murphy KG, *et al.* Actions of cocaine-and amphetamine-regulated transcript (CART) peptide on regulation of appetite and hypothalamo-pituitary axes *in vitro* and *in vivo* in male rats Brain Res. 2001; 893: 186-94.

[12] de Gortari P, Méndez M, Rodríguez-Keller I, Pérez-Martínez L, Joseph-Bravob P. Acute ethanol administration induces changes in TRH and proenkephalin expression in hypothalamic and limbic regions of rat brain. Neurochem Int. 2000; 37: 483-96.

[13] Amir S, Jackson IM. Immunological blockade of endogenous thyrotropin-releasing hormone impairs recovery from hyperglycemia in mice. Brain Res. 1988; 462: 160-2.

[14] Chen Y, Uemura K, Yoshioka S, *et al.* Centrally administered TRH-induced insulin secretion is impaired in the Otsuka-Long-Evans-Tokushima Fatty rats, a model of spontaneous non-insulin-dependent diabetes mellitus. J Auton Nerv Syst 1998; 71: 10-7.

[15] Rondeel JM, de Greef WJ, Heide R, Visser TJ. Hypothalamo-hypophysial-thyroid axis in streptozotocin-induced diabetes. Endocrinology 1992;130: 216-20.

[16] Ishiguro T, Iguchi A, Kunoh Y, *et al.* Relative contribution of nervous system and hormones to hyperglycemia induced by thyrotropin-releasing hormone in fed rats. Neuroendocrinology 1991; 54: 1-6.

[17] Amir S. Thyrotropin-releasing hormone (TRH) blocks glucagon-induced hyperglycemia in mice: dissociation of the antihyperglycemic and pituitary actions of TRH. Brain Res 1988; 455: 201-3.

[18] Roper MG, Qian WJ, Zhang BB, Kulkarni RN, Kahn CR, Kennedy RT. Effect of the insulin mimetic L-783,281 on intracellular Ca2+and insulin secretion from pancreatic beta-cells. Diabetes 2002; 51: S43-9.

[19] Maltese JY, Giraud P, Kowalski C, *et al.* Ontogenetic expression of peptidyl-glycine alpha-amidating monooxygenase mRNA in the rat pancreas. Biochem Biophys Res Commun 1989; 158: 244-50.

[20] Vara E, Idahl LA, Lindström P, Sehlin J, Tamarit-Rodriguez J. Insulin, glucagon, somatostatin, and thyrotropin-releasing hormone content and secretion by perifused fetal rat islets during culture. Acta Endocrinol (Copenh) 1990; 123: 353-8.

[21] Glasbrenner B, Malfertheiner P, Duntas L, Büchler M, Bereiter T, Ditschuneit H. Effects of TRH on pancreatic growth and secretion in rats. Pancreas 1990; 5: 37-41.

[22] Strbák V, Ouafik LH, Resetková E, *et al.* Thyrotropin releasing hormone in the pancreas of newborn rats from streptozotocin-treated mothers. Life Sci 1989; 44: 779-87.

[23] Yamada M, Shibusawa N, Hashida T, *et al.* Expression of thyrotropin-releasing hormone (TRH) receptor subtype 1 in mouse pancreatic islets and HIT-T15, an insulin-secreting clonal beta cell line. Life Sci 2000; 66:1119-25.

[24] Alhan E, Küçüktülü U, Erçin C, Efe H, Al S. The effects of calcium channel blocker and thyrotropin releasing hormone on acute necrotizing pancreatitis in rats. Res Exp Med (Berl) 1999; 199: 51-8.

[25] Luo LG, Yano N. Expression of thyrotropin-releasing hormone receptor in immortalized beta-cell lines and rat pancreas. J Endocrinol 2004; 181: 401-12.

[26] Doong ML, Yang H. Intravenous glucose infusion decreases intracisternal thyrotropin-releasing hormone induced vagal stimulation of gastric acid secretion in anesthetized rats. Neurosci Lett 2003; 340: 49-52.

[27] Pizzi M, Boroni F, Benarese M, Moraitis C, Memo M, Spano P. Neuroprotective effect of thyrotropin-releasing hormone against excitatory amino acid-induced cell death in hippocampal slices. Eur J Pharmacol 1999; 370: 133-7.

[28] Yano N, Luo L. Effect of thyrotropin releasing hormone (TRH) on gene expressions in rat pancreas: approach by microarray hybridization. JOP 2004; 5: 193-204.

[29] Buteau J, Foisy S, Rhodes CJ, Carpenter L, Biden TJ, Prentki M. Protein kinase Czeta activation mediates glucagon-like peptide-1-induced pancreatic beta-cell proliferation. Diabetes 2001; 50: 2237-43.

[30] Smith J, Yu R, Hinkle PM. Activation of MAPK by TRH requires clathrin-dependent endocytosis and PKC but not receptor interaction with beta-arrestin or receptor endocytosis. Mol Endocrinol 2001; 15:1539-48.

[31] Palomero T, Barros F, del Camino D, Viloria CG, de la Peña P. A G protein beta gamma dimer-mediated pathway contributes to mitogen-activated protein kinase activation by thyrotropin-releasing hormone receptors in transfected COS-7 cells. Mol Pharmacol 1998; 53: 613-22.

[32] Ohmichi M, Sawada T, Kanda Y, *et al*. Thyrotropin-releasing hormone stimulates MAP kinase activity in GH3 cells by divergent pathways. Evidence of a role for early tyrosine phosphorylation. J Biol Chem 1994; 269: 3783-8.

[33] Andreev J, Galisteo ML, Kranenburg O, *et al*. Src and Pyk2 mediate G-protein-coupled receptor activation of epidermal growth factor receptor (EGFR) but are not required for coupling to the mitogen-activated protein (MAP) kinase signaling cascade. J Biol Chem 2001; 276: 20130-5.

[34] Wang YH, Jue SF, Maurer RA. Thyrotropin-releasing hormone stimulates phosphorylation of the epidermal growth factor receptor in GH3 pituitary cells. Mol Endocrinol. 2000; 14: 1328-37.

[35] Luo L, Yano N, Luo JZ. The molecular mechanism of EGF receptor activation in pancreatic beta-cells by thyrotropin-releasing hormone. Am J Physiol Endocrinol Metab 2006; 290: E889-99.

[36] Cras-Méneur C, Elghazi L, Czernichow P, Scharfmann R. Epidermal growth factor increases undifferentiated pancreatic embryonic cells *in vitro*: a balance between proliferation and differentiation. Diabetes 2001; 50: 1571-9.

[37] Luo LG. International Society for stem cell research (ISSCR) 2nd Annual Meeting, Boston MA 2004; Abstract 183:147.

http://dx.doi.org/10.5772/57550

[38] Li Y, Hansotia T, Yusta B, Ris F, Halban PA, Drucker DJ. Glucagon-like peptide-1 receptor signaling modulates beta cell apoptosis. J Biol Chem 2003; 278: 471-8.

[39] Luo LG, Yano N, Jackson I. 86th Annual Endocrine Meeting 2004 New Orleans Louisana June 16-19. 2004; Abstract: OR 46-2, pp 141.